PRAISE FOR
YOGA FOR BETTER SLEEP

"With an in-depth presentation of the nature of sleep, Stephens orients the avid reader to what lies behind getting, or not getting, a good night's sleep, offering yoga practices—including yoga *nidra*—that are an exquisite means of self-enquiry and awakening. I hope this book find its way into the hands of many."

> —RICHARD MILLER, author of *Yoga Nidra* and cofounder of International Association of Yoga Therapists

"Finally, a yogic approach to insomnia that integrates yoga and science! Mark Stephens distills the essential insights of neuroscience, psychology, and the yoga tradition to better understand the nature of sleep and how to improve sleep using yoga rather than pharmaceutical drugs and narrow behaviorist techniques. With chapters on yoga for specific conditions—including stress, anxiety, and depression—and for different ages, this book offers an invaluable resource for anyone interested in better sleep and a healthier life.

> —DIANA ALSTAD, coauthor, with Joel Kramer, of
> *The Passionate Mind Revisited*

YOGA
FOR
BETTER
SLEEP

YOGA FOR BETTER SLEEP

ANCIENT WISDOM MEETS MODERN SCIENCE

Mark Stephens
Foreword by Sally Kempton

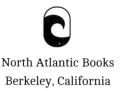

North Atlantic Books
Berkeley, California

Published by   Cover design by Deborah Berne
North Atlantic Books   Book design by Happenstance Type-O-Rama
Berkeley, California

Printed in the United States of America

Yoga for Better Sleep: Ancient Wisdom Meets Modern Science is sponsored and published by the Society for the Study of Native Arts and Sciences (dba North Atlantic Books), an educational nonprofit based in Berkeley, California, that collaborates with partners to develop cross-cultural perspectives, nurture holistic views of art, science, the humanities, and healing, and seed personal and global transformation by publishing work on the relationship of body, spirit, and nature.

North Atlantic Books' publications are available through most bookstores. For further information, visit our website at *www.northatlanticbooks.com* or call 800-733-3000.

Library of Congress Cataloging-in-Publication Data
Names: Stephens, Mark, 1958- author.

Title: Yoga for better sleep : ancient wisdom meets modern science / Mark
    Stephens.
Description: Berkeley, California : North Atlantic Books, [2019] | Includes
    bibliographical references and index.
Identifiers: LCCN 2018060951 (print) | LCCN 2019001675 (ebook) | ISBN
    9781623173647 (e-book) | ISBN 9781623173630 (paperback)
Subjects: LCSH: Sleep disorders—Alternative treatment. | Hatha yoga. | Mind
    and body. | BISAC: HEALTH & FITNESS / Sleep & Sleep Disorders. |
HEALTH &
    FITNESS / Yoga. | BODY, MIND & SPIRIT / Meditation.
Classification: LCC RC547 (ebook) | LCC RC547 .S734 2019 (print) | DDC
    613.7/046—dc23
LC record available at *https://lccn.loc.gov/2018060951*

1 2 3 4 5 6 7 8 9 KPC 24 23 22 21 20 19

Printed on recycled paper

For the sleepless:

May you have sweet dreams filled with magic.

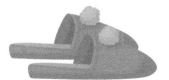

CONTENTS

Part II: Practices

FOREWORD

By Sally Kempton

Ever since I've known Mark Stephens, I've been impressed by the breadth of his knowledge of yoga. Not only is he a skillful and wise teacher, he's a true yoga adept, with deep knowledge of a range of practices, techniques, and philosophical approaches. So when he told me that he had written a book on yoga and sleep, I got excited. Why? Because I've been a longtime skeptic about whether yoga can help you sleep. I once spent ten years as a hard-core insomniac, a period when I rarely slept more than three or four hours a night. During those years I did a lot of yoga and meditation, and found that they could in many ways *substitute* for sleep. I could rest in Savasana, slipping in and out of *yoga nidra* and meditation, for five or six hours at a time, and get up with enough energy to get through a day. But I never found a posture or a series of postures or an approach to meditation that actually improved my ability to get into a "normal" sleep state, and stay there for seven or eight hours.

That's why I'm so grateful for what Mark has done in this book. Not only does he give us a clear, well-researched, and highly readable discourse on sleep science, he unpacks all the major varieties of insomnia and its causes. Most helpfully, he draws distinctions between the sleep issues of childhood and adolescence, the sleep issues of adulthood, and the problems of getting good sleep as we age.

But the real gold in this book is the fact that the practices and sequences Mark gives us really work, especially when you combine them with the other interventions he recommends. Mark never claims that one practice is the key. Instead, he shows you how to work with a range of techniques and ways to set up your sleeping situation, so that you gradually create a truly relaxing approach to bedtime.

I'm particularly grateful that he has organized the practice chapters according to the different categories of sleep disorder. There are *asanas* and breathing exercises that soothe hyperarousal, and practices for working with depression. There are sequences for teenagers and sequences for older people. Every chapter has a different balance of techniques and attitudes, aimed at helping individuals work with specific sleep issues. As I've been exploring them, I've been especially impressed by the ways they can be combined—and by Mark's expert understanding of how to combine them.

Yoga for Better Sleep is a sleep-resources library in itself. You'll find a full range of recommendations, from medical advice to meditation practices to *asana* and *pranayama,* to lifestyle hacks. Mark's instructions are clear and easy to follow—and granular enough so that you feel fully supported in both the techniques and the subtle attitudes that help the techniques take hold. I was particularly impacted by the sections on pranayama, which may inspire you to start experimenting with the range of breathing practices that can be adapted for both relaxing and self-energizing.

This is a book to keep by your bed, to practice with daily, and to use as a practice guide. I hope Mark's steady, comforting wisdom helps you create a sleep protocol you can live with. May it revolutionize your bedtime hours, and help you experience more and more deeply the true rest that we all need and deserve.

Sally Kempton is a meditation teacher, a contributing editor for *Yoga Journal,* and the author of *Meditation for the Love of It, Awakening Shakti,* and *Awakening to Kali.*

PREFACE

Sleep issues are among the greatest health and well-being concerns throughout the world. Often thought to be a problem largely isolated to the more industrialized Northern Hemisphere, sleep problems today are a global epidemic that extends to the underdeveloped nations in Africa, Asia, and Latin America.[1] The health, social, and economic consequences are vast, with increasing evidence that sleep problems are a partial cause and consequence of memory loss, learning problems, mood disorders, motor skill deficits, and mental health issues, all with potentially tragic effects. It is estimated that 50–70 million Americans suffer from sleep disorders, with around 10 million using prescription sleeping pills with disturbing psychological side effects.[2] We find similar rates of sleeping pill use in Europe, Japan, and other advanced industrialized societies.

While sleep medication helps many people, particularly when used in conjunction with sleep hygiene practices and psychological sleep therapies, there are promising alternatives found in ancient to modern yoga practices that are basically free, are available to all, and have few if any known side effects. Indeed, the primary side effect of yoga for better sleep is greater overall health, not "merely" better sleep.

Yet yoga is not a panacea for sleep disorders or any other health problem. Rather, yoga provides an effective complement to other practices, and taken together might be the best medicine.

Even as yoga has entered the cultural mainstream of most Western societies—witness yoga mats and yoga classes in films and advertisements wholly unrelated to yoga, such as selling cars or soft drinks—it remains a strange, weird, or socially unacceptable activity to millions of people. This is not surprising given the often esoteric and dogmatic ways that yoga is presented, and even less surprising when one scratches the historical surface of yoga to see or experience some of its ancient (and modern) practices. Superstitious beliefs, disproven philosophical and metaphysical assumptions, and bizarre self-mortification practices that are part and parcel of many of yoga's root sources are a major turnoff for many people.[3] Fortunately, yoga is evolving, including with the insights of modern culture and science, giving us theories and techniques that make sense and have proven benefits.

Yoga has always offered a diverse array of practices rooted in different philosophical foundations. In the past generation, it has diversified to the point of having such divergent ideas about yoga that some do not recognize the others as yoga. This trend has accelerated with many yoga styles branded and promoted as most original (does it matter?), most effective (for whom?), or otherwise best (a curious idea given that yoga is not about competition). As human interest would have it, most research into the efficacy of yoga in helping to heal ailments or promote well-being evaluates only the style of yoga favored by the researchers, such as Kundalini or Iyengar, or relatively obscure approaches such as Silverlight or Phoenix Rising. Even research conducted by noninterested researchers typically focuses on testing one style rather than posing the question of which yoga practices might be most effective in addressing a certain condition.

The aim of this book is to distill valid and practical yoga methods that are helpful in improving sleep. I consider a variety of traditional and innovative yoga practices in conjunction with the most recent neuroscience of sleep to better understand sleep problems and potential solutions. While I do not reject the use of prescription sleeping pills, which can be vitally important in some conditions, I recognize the overdependence on such sleep medications that are promoted as part of the survival strategy of large pharmaceutical companies, whose legal bottom-line responsibility is to their shareholders, not the well-being of humanity. Nor do I reject conventional psychological techniques such as cognitive behavioral therapy, an approach that has demonstrated significant success in improving sleep even as it is rooted in assumptions about the human mind and experience that can be reductionist and thereby can distort one's larger sense of self and greater depth that yoga aims to evoke.

To be clear, I do not recommend changing any doctor-prescribed medicines or other professionally prescribed practices without first discussing such decisions with one's doctor and other licensed health care providers, including mental health providers.

I do recommend exploring the safe options yoga offers. Here the focus is on basic and proven yoga practices, with primary attention given to breathing, meditation, and physical postures. In each of these areas, adaptive techniques are offered tailored to one's specific sleep issues, related health concerns, age, and other factors. I also point to insights from outside of yoga that are directly relevant to sleep, including sleep hygiene, diet, and other lifestyle choices.

Anyone and everyone can enjoy better sleep, which results in being more fully and consciously awake when not sleeping. *Yoga for Better Sleep* is designed for just this purpose.

Here is how to use this book:

- If you are interested in the science of sleep, the philosophy of yoga, and how the two meet, read part I before reading part II.

- If you have difficulty sleeping and do not know why, read part I. With greater insight into your sleep issues, choose the related chapters in part II for ways to have better sleep with yoga.

- If you are not interested in the science of sleep or the philosophy of yoga but simply want better sleep, reading part I will quickly put you to sleep!

- If you know why you have sleep issues, choose the related chapters in part II and the appendixes for ways to have better sleep with yoga.

If you want more detailed guidance with the postures, see *Yoga Adjustments: Philosophy, Principles, and Techniques,* and visit the Online Yoga Education section at *www.markstephensyoga.com.*

ACKNOWLEDGMENTS

The idea for this book arose in conversation with my sister, Melinda Stephens-Bukey. I am deeply grateful for her being a sounding board for my ideas, helping me focus on what is most important, and encouraging me to persist when questioning if writing this book was the best use of my energy in what seems a pretty crazy time in the world.

There are several others I thank:

Mike Rotkin for his advice on the organization of topics and for reading and critiquing the entire manuscript, making several critical suggestions on tone, style, and substance, and serving as a cameo model for chair yoga.

Jennifer Stanley, MD, for reading key chapters and offering her insights into sleep medicine while keeping me engaged on broader matters of the interrelations of medical science, spiritual being, and consciousness.

G. William Domhoff for sharing some of his unpublished work on dreams and the brain, helping me understand top-down versus bottom-up neuronal processes related to learning and memory, and helping me better understand the surprising political landscape of sleep science.

Sat Bir Singh Khalsa for his critique of the draft manuscript and related suggestions regarding the neurophysiology of sleep, the effects of sleep medication, and the role of cognitive behavioral therapy for insomnia.

Sally Kempton for years of heartfelt friendship and intelligent conversation about seemingly everything under the suns and moons of yoga, particularly for revealing how what is most powerful in yoga and life transcends words.

Ralph Quinn for guiding me on matters of depth psychology and encouraging me to keep looking forward even as some in the world tug in other directions.

Michael Stephens, my brother, for his active support in creating and maintaining the environment in which I could focus on my writing while offering me a deeper appreciation of the importance of living as close as possible to the rhythms of nature.

Diana Alstad for pointing me in the right direction on key sources and sharing her deep wisdom about sleep, life, and yoga.

Joel Kramer for inspiring me with his keen insights into yoga and life.

Anne Tharpe for her management savvy and her thoughtful observations on many topics covered in this book.

Dagmar Stuhr for bringing greater clarity, meaning, and joy to my life and work, for inspiring me to write more popular books, for her creative sensibilities that influenced the design of this book's cover, and for her delightful spirit that enriches everything inside.

Matthew Walker, Paul Glovinsky, Timothy McCall, MD, Roger Cole, Richard Miller, Eleanor Criswell, Gregg Jacobs, Rachel Manber, and Jason Ong helped me in various ways to better understand the nexus of sleep, the bodymind, and yoga.

Ray Charland, Sima Mehrbod, Mike Rotkin, and Rebecca Zabinsky graciously posed for the yoga posture photos in Part II.

Deep bows to the team at North Atlantic Books for expertly and kindly guiding the acquisition, editorial, design, publication, and distribution process, and for their commitment to diversity, social justice, and sharing relevant ideas.

Any errors are solely mine.

Lastly, a note on notes. Most books with yoga in the title do not provide bibliographic reference for the sources of their ideas and assertions. Although a blessing to the reader who might not care and, like me, identifies with Shakespeare's quip that "brevity is the soul of wit," this is unfortunate for the reader who wishes to know on whose shoulders the writer stands, whether there is supporting evidence for what is written, and where to go to further explore. While adding weight (and thus cost and encumbrance) to the book, my choice is to share with you the specific books, articles, correspondence, and conversations upon which my writing rests. Reading the endnotes will also help you fall asleep.

PART I

Foundations

We live in a world of diverse ideas about wellness and the practices that might best support living in the healthiest ways, including with better sleep. The scientific medical approach to sleep, which insists on evidence-based practices, is increasingly specialized and focused on reducing specific symptoms of sleep disorders. It is often very effective, yet equally often its solutions have significant unintended side effects, especially from prescription sleep medications.

Yoga takes a more holistic view of life and to healing what ails us, emphasizing personal lifestyle changes and ancient to modern techniques for improving our overall well-being. In recent years, the development of yoga into a mainstream cultural trend has brought it under a scientific lens. A growing body of evidence demonstrates that yoga can help in healing a variety of conditions, including some of the prime suspects—stress, anxiety, and depression—in insomnia and other sleep disorders.

To sleep better, we need to better understand the nature of sleep, which sleep science is doing, albeit with solutions that can be harmful and take us away from our true nature as whole beings. Yoga gives us better ways of understanding and living fully in our true nature. Bringing these odd bedfellows together offers much promise for better sleep, and with it, better lives.

Chapter

1

THE MYTHS AND NATURE OF SLEEP

Myth and Science

Sleep can be delightfully, curiously, even disturbingly mysterious, especially the last if sleep does not seem to come to you naturally, fully, or when you want it. We have only very recently come to closely understand its nature and purposes. This allows us to loosely define sleep as a state of altered consciousness coupled with physical inhibition in which we become largely separated from sensory experience, this even as we might experience wild, mundane, fantastic, yet often insightful dreams.

In the absence of this understanding, even with it, the mysteries of sleep have been the stuff of myth, typically given a dark hue in Western casts, just as we might expect of something that mostly happens in the night and in all its stillness can seem akin to death. It thus makes sense that the children of Nyx, the Greek goddess of the night, were Hypnos, the god of sleep, and Thanatos, the god of death, and that English poets from metaphysical Donne to romantic Shelley waxed on about the nexus of sleep and death. The adage "rest in peace" reflects this connection, even as it conveys an unintended meaning if wishing someone to have sweet dreams.

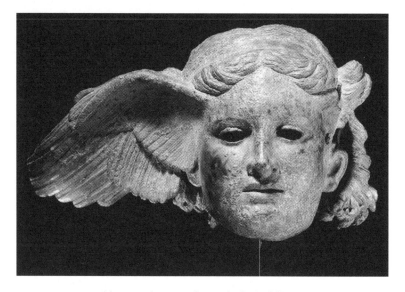

Hypnos, Ancient Greece's God of Sleep

We also find a mythologized view of sleep in ancient yogic thought, starting in the oldest known written source on yoga, *Rig Veda Samhita* (from around the fifteenth century BCE). There we learn of Ratri, the goddess of night, and her sister Ushas, goddess of the dawn and daughter of Lord Surya, the inestimably powerful sun god. From Ratri we get Navaratri, one of the great annual festivals in India, with nine nights celebrating the goddess Durga's slaying of "the demons of ego and greed," which, as we shall see, can play a part in sleep disorders.[1]

Ushas appears throughout the *Rig Veda* as a most revered god-dess for giving strength, dispelling darkness, and illuminating the true nature of the world, even if only regionally worshipped today in India during the festival of Chhath, which is all about giving thanks for light and the bounties of life.[2] We might wisely explore such themes.

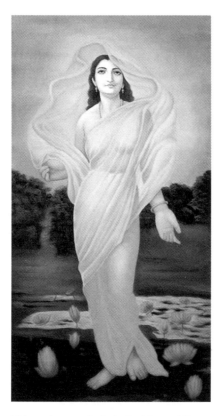

Ushas, Ancient India's Goddess of Dawn

These ancient myths often shaped rituals and other prac-tices, including yoga, that were intended to make life better, including Surya Namaskara, the early dawn bowing to the sun deity, Surya, in hope of his return to the sky each day.

In the most ancient yogic writings, the Vedas and Upanishads, we find recurring discussions of sleep as an expression or indication of different qualities of consciousness.[3] Various ancient to modern commentaries on these writings support often conflicting ideas about the nature of reality and consciousness, even as they all typically differentiate sleep, deep sleep, and awake states and the sensory conditions in each as reflections or sources of spiritual being. All recognize that consciousness changes in these states in relation to sensory awareness or nonawareness, anticipating discoveries in neuroscience and modern psychology of sleep-wake states and dreams.

We have learned more about the nature of sleep in the past generation than in the prior few millennia, helping to dispel myths in favor of reality.[4] Meanwhile, the art and science of yoga, including its understanding of personal psychology and practical, self-directed techniques for healthy living, has progressed more in the past two generations than since its origins some 3,500 years ago in the spiritual and superstitious mists of ancient India, generating more accessible, sensibly designed, and healthy practice techniques for improving life. Here we weave these strands of insight into a whole cloth of effective sleep strategies, integrating the insights and practices of yoga with those of sleep science to provide simple and effective tools for healthier sleeping and living, with less or no reliance on often harmful (if sometimes helpful) sleep medications.

Waking and the Awake State

From research in the modern laboratory, sleep and awake states are increasingly well understood using multiple electrical measurements and visual observations, what sleep scientists call polysomnography: electroencephalograph (EEG) for recording brain waves; functional magnetic resonance imaging (fMRI) for visually tracking brain activity; electromyograph (EMG) for evaluating nerve activity associated with movement in skeletal muscle; and electrooculograph (EOG) for detecting eye movement.[5] These precision technologies reveal the level and location of brain and other physical activity, allowing us to see, track, and measure what happens in the brain and elsewhere in the body during various stages and qualities of sleep, wake, drowsiness, quiet, and other nuanced states of consciousness and being.

When we are fully awake, our EEG rhythms have faster frequency and lower amplitude (think less vibration), with synchronized activity in small yet interrelated areas of the brain.[6] Neuroscientists refer to this as "low voltage fast activity," or LVFA. This enables us to do things like pay attention, remember, and be more consciously aware. When slower frequencies are more prevalent, we are quiet or drowsy. When waking and gradually transitioning to full wakefulness, we have increased prominence in (1) our low-amplitude beta/gamma rhythm (beta associated with normal waking consciousness, gamma with conscious attention), which stimulates simultaneous action across multiple neuronal areas, including light sensitivity; (2) our alpha rhythms (associated with a relaxed mental state), arousing the potential for conscious inner reflection; and (3) our theta rhythms (associated with active states), bringing about greater attention and memory.[7]

This transition into wakefulness originates in the brain stem through what neuroscientists call the ascending reticular activating system (ARAS).[8] Nerve fibers moving along a network of distinct dorsal and ventral pathways through multiple locations in the brain activate the forebrain, bringing us to a full wake state. We find a parallel "default network" active from the brain stem to the forebrain in humans when free of external environmental stimuli and thereby more engaged in purely inner awareness. This may identify what in yoga are called states of *pratyahara* and *dharana,* practices in which one relieves one's senses of external stimuli to open one's awareness to a meditative state and more pure consciousness.[9]

Intertwined with ARAS, several metabolic systems are at work in awakening us from sleep, led by rising serotonin, cortisol, norepinephrine, and histamine levels.[10] Soon compounds called hypocretins will excite the hypothalamus, helping to consolidate our wakefulness for the day. Taken together, our metabolic rate is rising, our sympathetic nervous system is activating, and we are getting full cortical (brain) arousal along with reawakened muscle tone.

The functional interaction between these calm yet wake-promoting elements of ARAS is mutually reinforcing. Their convergence—and their redundancy—is precisely why the normal human condition is to wake from sleep and remain in a wake state until other physiological forces and our behaviors cause sleepiness and sleep. We gradually slip into deepening sleep states and the surreal alternative world of dreams, this as the brain is doing its integrative magic.

Sleeping

It might seem as if sleep is a unitary state, even when punctuated by dreams, but it is nonetheless a varied state. Polysomnography reveals that when sleeping we have different combinations of EEG, fMRI, EMG, and EOG activity depending on the stage and quality of sleep. But before we get there, unless narcoleptic we must first become sleepy, and only then fall asleep. This occurs even when we resist it, as our body is conspiring to restore its energy, maintain its balance, and sustain its existence. The conspiracy involves two main players code-named Process S and Process C. Here is how they work together to generate and maintain sleep—interacting continuously—in what sleep scientist Alexander Borbély named the two-process model of sleep regulation.[11]

Process S: Natural Sleep Pressure

The longer we are awake, the more we feel the pressure to sleep. Sleep pressure results from a homeostatic control system (homeostasis is the state of steady internal conditions) that reflects the natural accumulation of sleep-inducing forces when awake, inhibiting the arousing effects of ARAS activity described above and of cortical neurons in the cerebral cortex—the gray matter of the brain where we think and take conscious action. Lacking this pressure, we would not have the pressure to sleep, causing imbalance in our overall physiological functioning (homeostasis).

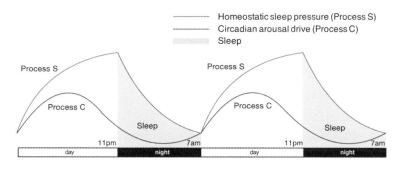

Process S and Process C

The main sleep chemical working to do this is adenosine, which connects the body's energy metabolism, brain activity, and sleep. The longer we are awake, the more adenosine levels rise in the forebrain.[12] As increased adenosine dampens the brain's nerve activity, we become sleepy. Even as one might wish to remain awake, this natural homeostatic control system is gradually yet steadily expressing an emphatic *no* as nitric oxide (NO) stimulates the release of the adenosine sleep force.[13] At the same time, prostaglandins and cytokines are introducing yet more potent sleep force.[14] The collective and accumulative effect of these homeostatic processes is the seeming magic of sleep.

When we fall asleep, these sources of sleep pressure are gradually and steadily relieved. Stay awake and the pressure increases. Yet strangely enough, if you pull an all-nighter, with sleep pressure building all through the wee hours, in the morning you get a second wind of energy, despite the increased homeostatic sleep drive. Why? Sleep-dependent Process S (dependent in that sleep pressure depends on how long you are asleep or awake) has just had a secret encounter with sleep-independent Process C.

Process C: Circadian Rhythm

Deep in our brain is a highly light-sensitive mechanism with a long name: the suprachiasmatic nucleus (fortunately, it is also called the SCN). The SCN is our master biological clock, controlling the timing, intensity, and duration of sleep through what is called circadian rhythm. (The term "circadian" was coined in the 1950s from the Latin *circa,* "around," and *dies,* "day.") While circadian rhythm controls the timing of biological processes in a variety of life forms, including plants, in humans it helps regulate our hormonal cycles, body temperature, appetite, and more—perhaps nothing more obviously than our daily sleep-wake cycle.[15] Relatively independently of Process S's homeostatic sleep drive, we tend to sleep and wake—and to feel sleep and wake tendencies even when awake—in sync with the cycle of day and night. Here is how it works.

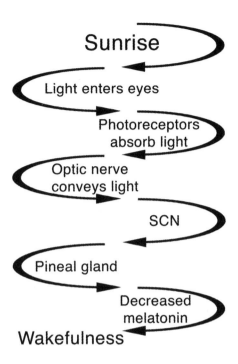

The Suprachiasmatic Nucleus

The SCN is our internal link to the natural twenty-four-hour daily light/dark cycle. It is located inside the hypothalamus, just above the optic chiasm, where optic nerves partially cross. Highly light-sensitive cells integrate environmental light data within the retina and send this information to the SCN. In turn, the SCN outputs this information through different pathways to stimulate hormone release and other timed physiological functions.[16]

One of these pathways is to the pineal gland, located deep in the center of the brain and long a subject of fantastic speculation in yogic, tantric, and Western medical and philosophical circles. The Greek physician, surgeon, and philosopher Galen

discovered the pineal gland around 170 CE, positing the presence of a "psychic pneuma" in nearby ventricles, leading some
of his contemporaries to run wildly with the idea that it is the
localized site of consciousness and/or the direct portal to the
divine. In his *Meditations on First Philosophy,* published in 1641,
the philosopher, mathematician, and scientist René Descartes
wrote about the relationship of body and soul, offering the
pineal gland as "the seat of the soul" (a change from earlier
views that it was in the chest).[17] Much later the pineal gland
became the third eye and the *ajna chakra,* never mentioned as
such in any pre-twentieth-century yogic or tantric source until
transliterated into such early sources in the late nineteenth
century by the quite imaginative Madame Blavatsky and other
Theosophists.[18]

While not nearly so romantic, the reality is that the pineal
gland is hardwired to the SCN, which contains our circadian
pacemaker, using the visually sourced light-based signals from
the SCN to time the release of melatonin.[19] Derived from serotonin, this hormone then naturally synchronizes our sleep-
wake patterns with the daily clock.[20] (The clock is slightly off: on
average its "day" is 24.2 hours, causing a slight drift toward later
sleep times every day, which most people address by sleeping
in on weekends.) Put differently, secretion of melatonin, which
is governed by the light-based clock of the SCN, synchronizes
our circadian rhythms. This makes Process C the regulatory
mechanism for sleep timing. Without it our sleep would fluctuate based solely on homeostatic sleep pressure, causing erratic
sleep patterns. Indeed, we know from travel across multiple
time zones as well as nighttime work schedules that disturbance
to our circadian rhythms wreaks havoc on our sleep.

When healthy and exposed to natural rhythms of daylight,
we are entrained to the sun, with Process S and Process C

working together to make it most natural for us to fall asleep a few hours after sunset and wake shortly after sunrise. As we will see, this dynamic is easily disturbed by everything from latitude-based seasonal light changes to caffeine to stress to travel to hormonal changes, to say nothing of shift work, leading to sleep disturbances, which in turn can cause or exacerbate many health problems. It can also be disturbed by a vast range of genetic defects and pathological conditions. In healthy functioning, these dynamic processes naturally bring us into the potentially nourishing, enlightening, and restorative worlds of different sleep states.

Sleep States

Our basic states are threefold: (1) wakefulness, (2) rapid eye movement (REM) sleep, and (3) non-rapid eye movement (NREM) sleep. Wakefulness was discussed above, and we revisit it in chapter 2. REM was discovered almost by accident in 1951 by a graduate student named Eugene Aserinsky in a University of Chicago physiology lab where he had hooked up his young son to an antiquated brain wave detector called the Offner Dynograph. After many hours of his son sleeping, Aserinsky heard the back-and-forth scribbling of the Dynograph's pens, which were registering both wake-like brain waves and eye movement. Because of the eye movement he thought his son was awake. Instead he discovered something hiding in plain view of all who had closely observed sleepers in the period before waking: rapid eye movement, or REM. Although Aserinsky noted this observation in a short article cowritten with his adviser, it was his fellow graduate student William Dement, with an interest in psychiatry and dreams, who pursued deeper research on it, eventually becoming a leading authority on sleep.[21]

Dement found that during most sleep, there is no REM. Being a rational scientist, he called this phase of sleep non-rapid eye movement, or NREM, which is where we spend most of our time when asleep. In healthy sleep, our physiological systems cycle between different stages of NREM sleep (light to deep to light to deep to …) and REM sleep, each of which has distinct characteristics and benefits, the disturbance of which can cause mild to severe health problems, including dementia. Since NREM temporally precedes REM, we first look at NREM.

NREM Sleep States

In NREM sleep, we gradually slip in and out of the deepest, quietest, most still, and restorative stages of sleep. With the onset of sleep, the wakeful LVFA EEG readings discussed earlier change to slow but high-amp waves, reflecting our drop into NREM, or slow-wave sleep.[22] Now the awakening neurons in the ARAS are quieting down as our homeostatic sleep forces (adenosine being the most powerful) are having their way. One's depth of sleep is also detected by how much noise it takes to wake a sleeping person. We move through four stages of NREM sleep (N1–N4), from light to deep, each signified by changes in brain wave activity.[23]

- N1: This is the transition between wakefulness and sleep. With theta activity in frontal sites we are still faintly aware of external sensory stimuli, yet with alpha activity in posterior sites we are utterly still. We are technically asleep but very easily roused. About half of all sleepers will say they were not asleep when roused from N1. This state is akin to *yoga nidra,* or lucid sleeping, first described in the ancient *Mandukya Upanishad* around 500 BCE as one of four states of consciousness (discussed below). Yoga nidra as a defined practice was popularized in the twentieth century by Swami Satyananda Saraswati and is widely taught today as a means of meditation and deep relaxation.[24]

- N2: This is full sleep onset. Sudden brain wave bursts called sleep spindles (they look like spindles on a printed EEG) alternate with large waves called K-complexes. We are slipping further into a nonconscious state where procedural learning—inaccessible to conscious recollection—may be occurring. Lasting on average only about ten to twenty-five minutes, the higher-amp, slower waves of N3 are beginning to manifest. We are not so easily roused, with around 85 percent of sleepers saying they were asleep once awakened from this state.

- N3: We are moving into deep sleep, also called slow-wave sleep (SWS). Sleep spindles and K-complexes are still present even as body temperature and heart rate drop and the brain begins using less energy. Now there are prominent high-amp but slow brain waves, with the delta waves of deep sleep becoming increasingly prominent. Our skeletal muscle tone is very low. We are still and quiet, even as we have slow rolling eye movements (SREMs), and tend to be in this state and the deeper delta state of N4 for up to around forty minutes. It takes significant external stimulation to be awakened (also in N4), and the awakened sleeper will report having been asleep.

- N4: The deepest sleep state. EEGs show delta and slow oscillations in the cerebral cortex and thalamus, signifying the deepest stilling interaction between the two hemispheres of the cortex.[25] Difficulty in differentiating N3 and N4 has led some sleep scientists to merge them into N3, or SWS.

REM Sleep State

Now comes the fantastic, sometimes fun, sometimes disturbing, seemingly delusional and hallucinatory state of sleep. Although we dream a little in NREM sleep, dreaming almost always occurs during REM sleep, as is known from asking sleepers who have been awakened out of this state as well as from EEGs, whether in brief REM episodes that punctuate NREM or longer REM sleep before awakening in the morning.[26] This was discovered in the early 1950s by those pioneering graduate students in Chicago and their professor, Nathaniel Kleitman, using EEG and EMG (measuring muscle tone) to detect and describe a constellation of tonic and phasic episodes.[27]

Twenty-first-century neuroscientists and research psychologists are now discovering in tremendous detail what is happening in the brain and elsewhere in the body during REM sleep, even closing in on the sources, meaning, and content of dreams. These discoveries are part of deeper research into the nature of REM sleep, including mapping neuronal processes of REM, how they are controlled, and how REM is related to memory and learning.[28]

The ARAS pathways that we saw earlier causing us to wake and stay awake are also activated in REM sleep, but with the brain stem under hypothalamic control.[29] This area of the brain is highly involved in emotion, memory, and intuition, and possibly in consolidating daily lived experience for long-term recollection.[30] Theta waves are becoming dominant, as during meditation, which we discuss in chapter 3. Along with this theta activity, ponto-geniculo-occipital (PGO) waves are thought to be bringing visual and cognitive dream imagery into our awareness.[31] And there is much more going on.

Table 1.1. REM and NREM Sleep

SLEEP ACTIVITY	REM	NREM
Eye movement	Rapid	Slow
Body movement	Muscle twitches	Muscle relaxation
Vital signs	Fluctuating	Stable
Muscle tone	Decreased	Some in skeletal muscles
Dreams	Common	Rare
Sexual organs	Commonly excited	Rarely excited
EEG	Low voltage	Slow waves, spindles, V-waves, K-complexes
Percent of time asleep—adults	20–25	75–80
Percent of time asleep—infants	50	50

Soon after the discovery of REM, Michel Jouvet discovered "paradoxical sleep" in which the EEG indicates one is in a wake state yet skeletal muscle is essentially paralyzed, what is called muscle atonia.[32] Muscle atonia is one of the most definitive features of REM sleep, and both beneficial and potentially problematic.[33] The benefit is that we are mostly still when sleeping and dreaming. Muscle atonia becomes problematic only when it occurs with some sleep disorders, such as when someone with narcolepsy collapses as they suddenly fall asleep while standing, or conversely, in the disturbance of muscle atonia when someone with REM sleep behavior disorder (RBD) physically acts out their dreams, and in conditions such as bruxism (grinding the teeth when sleeping), sleepwalking during NREM sleep, and sexsomnia (automated sexual behavior while sleeping).[34] (These and other parasomnias are discussed in chapter 2.) Even amid muscle atonia, REM sleep in most adults is characterized by penile erection in sexually healthy and potent males and increased vaginal blood pressure in females, with neither of these related to sexsomnia but rather entirely normal.[35]

Throughout our sleep, we cycle repeatedly through the various NREM and REM states on average five times, with each cycle lasting about ninety minutes. When we first fall asleep, we come into light NREM, gradually progress to deeper NREM, then momentarily have a REM episode. In REM episodes, we are often briefly or even fully awakened. Except in pathological conditions such as narcolepsy, the sleep architecture (basic structural organization of our sleep into NREM and REM states) given by these cycles begins with light NREM, which progressively deepens, waxes, and wanes, concluding with REM. This alternation between NREM and REM throughout our sleep is thought to be caused by REM on/off neurons reciprocally interacting to shift our cycle, with REM episodes increasing and NREM decreasing over the course of our sleep.[36] While on/off neurons arising from the brain stem are primarily involved in NREM-REM cycles, there are several other contributing factors, including stress, emotion, temperature, light, and homeostatic forces.[37]

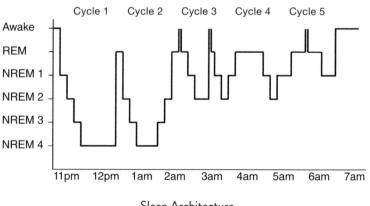

Sleep Architecture

Meanwhile, we dream, mostly during REM sleep, which is the likely reason most people have heard of REM but not NREM. Dreams have fascinated, bewildered, entertained, frightened, and enlightened humankind since the origins of consciousness. They have been the stuff of imagination, myth, creative intellectual speculation, and deep intellectual and scientific exploration everywhere in the world. Modern psychiatry and psychology, starting with Sigmund Freud's *The Interpretation of Dreams* in 1899, has attempted to systematically relate dreams to repressed emotion and thought. Carl Jung offered that dreams are symbolic messages from one's deeper being that suggest areas for deeper self-reflection, whereas the holistic Gestalt therapist Fritz Perls sought to elicit everything that appears in one's dreams as potential portals of insight into one's entire personality.[38] Dream study among psychological researchers continues to progress, increasingly with the tools of neuroscience.[39]

Dreams are activated by impulses from the brain stem mentioned above in discussing REM states, stimulating visual and movement areas of the brain, while brain areas involved in emotion and memory (the hippocampus and amygdala) are also active and possibly involved in the integration of our memories. It is thought that experiences of running, being unable to run, floating, and other such physical-action-related dream impressions arise from these interconnected areas occurring amid muscle atonia.

Rather than dreams reflecting hidden emotions or motives, much of sleep science is pointing to dreams as motivationally neutral, the only meaning in them being the meaning we later consciously bring to them. Another view is that during REM sleep we are unraveling and integrating emotionally significant experiences and altering and integrating daily learning, even if dreaming does not necessarily depend upon motivationally relevant stimulation.[40] Whether dreams reflect inner drives remains a hot topic in sleep science and psychology.

States of Consciousness in Ancient Yoga

It is tempting to neatly associate our sleep stages, their cycles, and our dream states as identified in neuroscience with the ideas about wake, sleep, and dream states found in ancient yoga texts. After all, both are attempting to describe states of consciousness, albeit one using primarily the scientific method that marshals verifiable and replicable evidence, the other a quasi-phenomenological method of reflection on experience, observation of others, and creative interpretation of those insights along with far-ranging imaginative ideas.[41]

To be clear, most ancient yoga writings are primarily interested in liberation from conditions of suffering, what is most often considered a spiritual malaise. Thus, as we consider yogic perspectives on sleep, wake, dreams, and consciousness, it behooves us to appreciate that the motivation in these writings is not about establishing scientific fact. Yet within these conversations (early yoga writings were very much considered to be intelligent exchanges), we can find insights that the finest nets of science often miss and that complement scientific insights. In the end, what we are primarily interested in here is understanding and improving sleep as a means of greater well-being, regardless of the source or method that informs us.

While some of the states of consciousness ancient yogis describe might seem akin to sleep stages, as noted earlier with respect to the lightest stage of NREM sleep and yoga nidra, in making this association one would be not only overstretching what we understand as fact but overstretching what is written in ancient texts. Stages or cycles are nowhere to be found in the ancient yogic literature in specific reference to sleep, only in reference to consciousness itself, with each state bringing one successively along a path that is no longer caught up in the realm of outer things or inner conflict, but in the assumed original unity of the mind or universe (which are often thought to be the same).

In some of the earliest yoga sources, we can find discussion of differentiated states of consciousness, most clearly in the *Mandukya Upanishad* (cited earlier), a primary source of nondualist Advaita Vedanta philosophy from around the fifth century BCE.[42] The self is said to consist of four *padas* (foundations), each representative or expressive of our four states of consciousness.

- *Vaiśvānara,* "Of all men" (or, now, people): the waking state. Consciousness is turned outward through seven "limbs" (head, eyes, mouth, ears, lungs, stomach, feet) and nineteen "mouths" (the five sense organs, five organs of action, five qualities of breath [*prana vayus*], mind, intellect, thought, and sense of one's personal self).

- *Taijasa,* "Of light": the dream state. Consciousness is turned inward through the same pathways given for the waking state, but with more subtlety.

- *Prājña,* "Of knowledge": the deep dream state, with a quality of *prājñāna,* "knowing."

- The fourth pada is unnamed, "measureless," nondual, in the original unity of consciousness, of the universe.

From close reading of this and other ancient sources on yoga and sleep, including the other principal Upanishads, *Brahmasūtra, Bhagavadgitā,* and the early fourth century CE *Yoga Sūtra of Patañjali,* beginning in the late twentieth century the most oft-cited work of yoga philosophy, we never find deep

inquiry into the nature of either the dream state or deep sleep.[43]
Contemporary yoga teachings, drawing heavily from Western
psychology, do inquire more deeply about stages of sleep and
consciousness, particularly regarding yoga nidra practices.[44]
Where we do find discussion of dreams, they are often seen as
a more refined quality of consciousness than the full waking
state, and the deep dream state closer yet to pure knowing consciousness as we move away from sensory awareness. This is
a curious notion given that our clearest consciousness might
come about not in the delusional states we experience in dreams
but in being fully awake with our senses attuned to all they can
absorb. It is a more tantric sensibility that we also find in some
contemporary yoga that is open to the fullest exploration of
mindfulness, psychosomatics, embodied consciousness, and life
in the here and now, central themes we will soon explore in
cultivating good sleep.

The Purpose of Sleep

Sleep is part of nature's insistence upon nourishing and rein-
tegrating the brain and restoring our bodies for everything we
do and experience when awake. Whereas yogis might emphasize how sleep can help balance our *gunas*—our innate qualities
of energy, inertia, and harmony—and open us to clearer consciousness, neuroscientists and others involved in sleep science
are looking very closely and with increasing precision at neurological and physiological processes in sleep, wake, and transitional states. We now have a better understanding of why we
sleep than ever before.

When sleeping we are not merely not awake. Instead, our
sleep state is "an exquisitely complex, metabolically active, and
deliberately ordered series of unique stages" during which we

restore our capacities to be fully and clearly conscious and functional when awake.[45] It is increasingly clear that sleep is the fundamental foundation of all aspects of our health, with fateful effects on metabolism, immunity, memory, learning, creativity, nutrition, mood, emotion, motor skills, and overall physiological function throughout life. The body is rebuilding and restoring its tissues and optimizing its interrelated physiological systems—cognitive, cardiovascular, endocrine, musculoskeletal, respiratory, digestive, urinary, and reproductive.

We need only reflect on a poor night of sleep to personally appreciate its effect on basic functions such as clear thinking, decision making, steady mood, stamina, and coordination. Yet even when we might not experience diminished capacities for healthy living, sometimes thinking we are just fine with five or six hours of sleep, the reality is that we are deceiving and harming ourselves. Unless you have an extremely rare gene found in a very tiny percentage of humans, you need around seven or eight hours of sleep to be healthy, with need defined not by your subjective experience, which is often disguised by stimulants such as coffee, tea, and other caffeinated drinks, but "whether or not that amount of sleep is sufficient to accomplish all that sleep does."[46]

The primary purposes of sleep are restoration of brain functions affecting four main areas of daily life:

- **Ability to think clearly and with focused attention.**[47] It appears that sleep disturbance in otherwise healthy people impairs the prefrontal cortex, the nerve pathways leading to it, and the posterior parietal cortex, which is directly connected to the prefrontal cortex, where we actively think.[48] High-frequency oscillations needed for cortical function are impaired, basal forebrain projections are inhibited and impact visual attention and responsiveness to new experiences, and optimal dopamine levels are altered, causing weakened cognitive function.

- **Ability to integrate new information (i.e., learn) and recall what we have learned (memory).**[49] Several related mechanisms can be affected by sleep disturbance or deprivation, including hormonal stress response to disrupted sleep, causing adrenal stress corticosterone levels to rise and consequently inhibiting the hippocampal neurogenesis that is required for full cognitive restoration during sleep. Sleep disruption can also affect memory by disturbing synaptic homeostasis during NREM sleep and inhibiting the consolidation and stabilization of unstable memories that might otherwise be too easily aroused and freely expressed (i.e., labile).[50]

- **Emotional balance and flexibility.**[51] Most of us know from personal experience that we are moodier after a poor night of sleep. Neuroscience is getting closer to explaining why sleep deprivation makes us more reactive to negative experiences, why our facial expressions are compromised, and why it is more difficult to accurately interpret others' emotions: emotional memory and our mesolimbic reward networks (which lead us to gravitate toward or resist things) that are nourished in normal REM sleep are impaired when that sleep is disturbed. "Keep dreaming" should not get such a bad rap, especially given how disrupted sleep plays into fear and anxiety.

- **Optimal motor skills, such as walking along a serpentine path or balancing on our feet or hands.**[52] In a seminal study conducted in Harvard University's neurophysiology lab in the early 2000s, sleep researchers found strong evidence for brain-state-dependent motor skill development, including relationships between sleep stage and task complexity, with complex skills more dependent on REM sleep and simple tasks more dependent on NREM stage N2 sleep.[53]

Alzheimer's Disease and Brain Cleansing

Looking more closely at sleep and cognitive dysfunction, we find increasing evidence that sleep disturbance and deprivation are associated with dementia, including Alzheimer's disease. Alzheimer's disease is a chronic and progressive neurological disorder involving cognitive and functional disability; it causes most cases of dementia.[54] Part of the insidious nature of Alzheimer's is its quiet yet gradual and persistent manifestation, which worsens over time.[55] The pathophysiological process of Alzheimer's begins to develop prior to experiencing the mild cognitive impairment that defines its earliest diagnosed stage. Although genetic factors appear significant in many cases of Alzheimer's, the causes remain largely mystifying, this despite billions of dollars of research into its etiology and pathophysiology.

Some of the most promising research into the causes of Alzheimer's is related to plaque accumulation in beta-amyloid and tau protein synthesis that appears in certain parts of the brain. (Beta-amyloid normally plays an essential role in neural growth and repair, and tau protein normally stabilizes microtubules that are essential in cellular processes.) Neuroscientist and sleep psychologist Matthew Walker recognized these areas as the very parts of the brain that generate NREM sleep, which is disturbed in people with Alzheimer's. Walker collaboratively investigated this with William Jagust, a leading Alzheimer's researcher, discovering that "the disruption of deep NREM sleep was … a hidden middleman brokering the bad deal between amyloid and memory impairment in Alzheimer's disease."[56]

This left the question of whether the loss of deep sleep might cause beta-amyloid plaque accumulation. Posed differently: what, if any, role does deep sleep play in clearing plaque from the brain? The answer came to Walker and Jagust through the contemporaneous research of Maiken Nedergaard, who discovered that neural cleansing tremendously increases during deep NREM sleep, including the removal of debris from the glial cells that surround neurons.[57] This "glymphatic system" (coined in relation to the lymphatic system that removes interstitial debris from tissues elsewhere in the body) literally cleans the brain, including accumulated plaque from beta-amyloid and tau protein synthesis.

Plaque accumulation occurs over the lifespan. Sleep is a daily opportunity. The primary preventive practice for diminishing the loss of brain function, including memory, is healthy sleep throughout life. Every little bit of deep sleep helps. If you are interested in helping to ensure you have the healthiest possible mind as you develop and age, it makes plain sense to do all you reasonably can to sleep as well as you can, to sleep yourself into greater wellness.

If a stronger clearer mind, increased memory, more balanced emotions, and increased physical function are not enough to motivate one to sleep well, consider additional restorative and wellness benefits. Sleeping well enhances overall immune function, helping to keep us from getting sick, helping us heal when ailing, even helping to heal physical wounds. It reduces the incidence of cardiovascular disease. It promotes more balanced hormones, including those that play a role in metabolism. It promotes human growth hormone in adult men. And it simply feels good.

In recent years, neuroscientists, medical scientists, and both research and clinical psychologists have made tremendous strides in understanding the causes and consequences of sleep disturbances, some of which we have briefly explored. They have made significant contributions to helping people sleep better, primarily with the assistance of medication, cognitive behavioral therapy, and sleep hygiene strategies that we discuss in chapter 3. In the next chapter, we look more closely at sleep disturbance, including different types of insomnia, sleep apnea, and what in yoga parlance are called *kleshas* (mental disturbances), *samskaras* (deeply ingrained mental-behavioral patterns), and the *gunatrayas* (energetic tendencies). In doing so, we gain deeper and clearer insight into our own sleep problems.

Chapter

2

THE NATURE OF SLEEP DISORDERS

Most of us have experienced poor sleep. Tossing and turning not merely in our bed but in our mind, sleep creeps further away, or comes and goes throughout the night. Sleeping in fragmented bits, never getting deep or nourishing restoration, we finally rise only to feel mentally and physically fatigued or disoriented. Whether persistent or periodic, stress-related or not, the effects are largely the same: we move through our waking life feeling tired, moody, out of sync—sometimes so off-kilter that we do not recognize that we are sleep deprived, or we disguise our condition with caffeine, other substances, or unhealthy eating. If this sounds familiar, know you are far from alone—and know you can sleep better using proven healthy sleep practices.

In reflecting on our sleep, there is a tendency to think about how long we slept more than how well. Quantity and quality are both important. For many years, I slept about six hours per night.

Some nights I had difficulty falling asleep, or woke in the middle of the night and stayed awake for what could seem like an eternity, or woke well before the crack of dawn knowing I needed more sleep yet no less wide awake. Despite these far less than optimal experiences, I usually felt plenty of energy throughout the day, especially because I started the day with the perfect cappuccino, green tea, or some other caffeinated drink, exactly what my relatively energetic nature desired. Other times I fell into the common midafternoon energy slump, sometimes taking a nap, other times taking a shot of espresso or drinking tea. (Tea leaves have more caffeine than coffee beans, but tea's caffeine is somewhat diluted with long brewing.) Nonetheless, I felt okay, even a sense of luck in being able to function well on as little as five hours of sleep, accomplishing lots of work and having plenty of energy for vigorous exercise.

Little did I know I was fooling myself: extensive sleep research, discussed in chapter 1, shows conclusively that most of us need around seven to eight hours of sleep per night.[1] Before discussing the consequences of inadequate sleep, many of which are suggested in what we covered in the previous chapter regarding the purposes of sleep, we first consider the nature and causes of sleep disturbance and deprivation. We begin with the dominant medical and behaviorist models before presenting a more humanistic, phenomenological, and existentialist view that expands and refines the yoga perspective.

Sleep and Wakefulness Disorders

Problems with sleep are not merely or narrowly sleep disorders, but often quality or balance of life issues, or other health problems, that lead to and are typically exacerbated by sleep issues. This makes it important to consider the whole person and one's larger lifestyle in understanding difficulties with sleep.

Thus, even the title of this section is somewhat problematic as it might imply that sleep and wakefulness disorders are separate, which, given that we are whole beings, they are not. Although this might seem like an insignificantly small detail, successful sleep practices reveal its importance.

The world's leading sleep research organizations (American Academy of Sleep Medicine, European Sleep Research Society, Japanese Society of Sleep Research, and Latin American Sleep Society) have collaboratively produced the *International Classification of Sleep Disorders* (ICSD), presently in its third edition (2014). Its two most significant sleep disorder diagnoses are insomnia and sleep-related breathing disorders.[2] (See appendix I for all sixty diagnoses, some of which are covered in this chapter. Sleep disorders identified in the *Diagnostic and Statistical Manual of Mental Disorders,* fifth edition [*DSM-V*] are closely aligned with those of the *ICSD.*) All were developed within a biological model of psychiatry, which, as we will see, can be as problematic as it is insightful.

Here we tour and briefly visit different types of insomnia and other sleep disorders along with their known causes and associations, including stress, anxiety, depression, pain, fatigue, obesity, neurological problems, and timing issues that include age, hormones, circadian disturbance, chronotypes, jet lag, shift work, and drugs, including the ones you might very much enjoy, without knowing how they can disturb your sleep and cause an array of health problems.

Insomnia

Insomnia is the most common sleep disorder, found among about 30–35 percent or more of the adult population (at least 50 percent complain of occasional insomnia), with 6–10 percent meeting the criteria for chronic insomnia, while those

over fifty years of age and women have higher rates of insomnia than younger people and men.[3] It is also perhaps the most
commonly misunderstood and misperceived sleep disorder, as
some people think they slept poorly (due to prior experience
with poor sleep) while testing reveals they slept just fine.[4] Until
recently, insomnia was differentiated as primary insomnia (not
caused by a comorbidity) or secondary insomnia (caused by
and typically exacerbating a comorbidity), distinctions that have
faded in favor of the more specific classification of sleep disorders reflected in the *ICSD*.

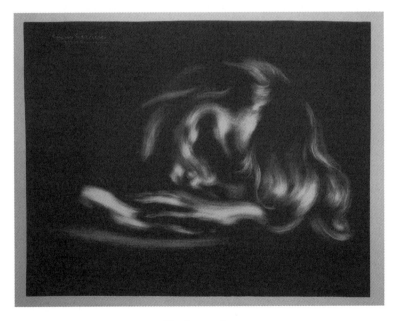

The Insomniac

If you can sleep but do not give yourself the rich and effective opportunity to do so, you do not have insomnia. If you
give yourself the opportunity to sleep but cannot get adequate
sleep, you have some form of insomnia, whether associated

with another condition or not. Impaired daytime functioning is another general trait of insomnia.

Short-term insomnia is characterized by difficulty initiating sleep, difficulty staying asleep, and/or waking earlier than desired, along with daytime symptoms at least a few times per week for less than three months. Once awake, you feel unrefreshed or fatigued or have difficulty concentrating, more easily experience mood disturbances, have impaired performance at work or in school, have greater behavioral difficulties, are more prone to making mistakes and having accidents, and ruminate a lot about your dissatisfaction with sleep. You also cannot completely explain these difficulties by not having enough time allotted to sleep or by being in a place that is noisy, where you feel unsafe, or that is otherwise physically distracting or uncomfortable, nor by having some other sleep disorder such as sleep apnea or restless legs syndrome. Short-term insomnia is also short-term, meaning less than three months in duration.

We can have short-term insomnia due to a variety of causes (discussed in some detail below): pain, stress, stimulants such as caffeine or nicotine, and sedatives such as alcohol (first it stimulates you, then it sedates you to sleep, then after a few hours the sedation wears off and you wake up).

Chronic insomnia has all the characteristics of short-term insomnia plus two highly significant differences: (1) it is chronic, and (2) it is almost invariably caused or precipitated by one or more identifiable factors that are not short-term event related, discussed below.

Other insomnia disorders have some but not all of the symptoms and characteristics described above for short-term insomnia—not daytime consequences—but are usually associated with either too much time in bed (more than nine hours) or too little (less than six hours and thinking it is okay because you feel okay).

Each of these types of insomnia can involve either sleep *onset* difficulty or sleep *maintenance* difficulty, or both. In sleep onset insomnia, we have difficulty falling asleep; in sleep maintenance insomnia, we have difficulty staying asleep, especially if we have awakened in the early morning before getting a healthy quantity of sleep.

What Causes Insomnia

There are many possible causes of insomnia in any given person, causes that can be and often are interrelated. Here we will look at the leading causes, including stress and anxiety, hyperarousal and depression, physical pain and fatigue, timing and energetic imbalances, and the influence of drugs, ranging from alcohol and nicotine to some prescription medications and strains of marijuana, rooting our observations in the insights of yoga, neurobiology, and psychology to highlight the forces that manifest and mediate insomnia.[5]

Stress, Anxiety, PTSD, and Hyperarousal

There is a relatively new turn of phrase we hear daily in nearly every walk of life: "no worries" or "no problem." It is often used in place of what in past years might have been "of course" or "I would be happy to." It signifies that worry is part of daily life. Worry is also a common feature of insomnia as it brings us to rumination, which leads to greater stress, anxiety, and hyperarousal.

Many emotional and psychological conditions are interrelated, including stress and anxiety, and can have varying levels of intensity. Although a low level of stress might help with motivation or adaptation to things in life, increased stress can interfere with concentration, make us more irritable, and interfere with sleep, whereas high levels of stress can cause acute or chronic insomnia and lead to cardiovascular disease, ulcers, and other serious health problems. Chronic stress makes us increasingly anxious and can lead to a generalized anxiety disorder in which our stress and worry are irrationally out of proportion to the reality of our situation, with palpable symptoms such as short-ness of breath, rapid heart rate, muscular tension, fatigue, and greater restlessness. These escalating conditions of stress and anxiety can directly cause sleep onset insomnia and sleep main-tenance insomnia, which in turn exacerbate stress, anxiety, and other mental health problems.[6]

Even when stress is not chronic, a stressful day can lead to an evening of obsessive rumination on the events that caused the stress, leading us into a state of hyperarousal, more popularly known as the fight-or-flight response. Hyperarousal also arises from being triggered in relation to long-term, deeply held trau-matic experiences, whether from car accidents, assaults, natural disasters, or other traumas, and is a diagnostic criterion for post-traumatic stress disorder (PTSD).[7]

Hyperarousal is expressed physiologically by activation of our sympathetic nervous system, the release of the neurotrans-mitter norepinephrine in the brain, and an adrenal response that causes the release of adrenaline and cortisol. As a result, our heart races, we breathe more quickly, our muscular tension increases, we become more focused and hypervigilant, and we are thereby better prepared to act in response to a threatening situation. Among those with PTSD, there is also an increasing likelihood of deeply disturbing and frightening nightmares, which in turn makes it scary to go to sleep, even more so with complex post-traumatic stress disorder (C-PTSD), which is most associated with an extended period of childhood physical or sexual abuse.[8] Although the sympathetic nervous system response can save our life, it can also cause overreaction and place us in greater danger. Hyperarousal exacerbates sleep disorders as the activation of the sympathetic nervous system fully revs us, making it difficult to settle down and sleep.[9]

Depression

Depression is a common emotional condition, and, like stress, when mild it can lead to deeper self-reflection or calling attention to oneself for the support of others. It is often associated with stress and anxiety, but also happens independently of those states. It is interwoven with the whole of our lives and can arise in natural reaction to a vast range of life events such as an adverse childhood, relationship issues, loss, finances, menopause, injury and illness, substance abuse, and an array of psychiatric disorders.[10] These causes as well as one's larger life situation give rise to a vast range of depressive states, from melancholy to major depressive disorder (MDD).

All types of depression are interdependent, to varying degrees, with sleep quality, but not necessarily in the ways one might expect. There are seemingly contradictory tendencies. With depression (especially MDD), there is typically sleep disturbance, and not only when one is both depressed and manic (bipolar disorder). Perhaps it is the inherent isolation and darkness of sleep that can make it elusive or fragmented to those experiencing depression. Although acute sleep deprivation has long proven effective as a powerful antidepressant treatment,[11] light deprivation, which disturbs our circadian clock, is also associated with depression, including seasonal affective disorder (even as there is no evidence of seasonal variation in mild forms of depression).[12]

Despite the seemingly contrary findings, we generally find that depression and sleep issues are in bed together (comorbid), and there is increasing evidence that healthy sleep contributes to a brighter outlook on life, as we explore in the next chapter.[13]

Physical Pain and Fatigue

Anyone who has had a headache or painful physical injury can attest to how pain can disturb sleep onset and maintenance, with intense pain sometimes making it impossible to sleep without medication. Several studies chronicle the relationship between pain and insomnia, with the greatest attention given to chronic pain.[14] Chronic pain makes it more difficult to initiate sleep, more difficult to have undisturbed sleep, more likely to wake up too early, and more likely that one's sleep is not restorative, which gains salience when we appreciate that about 40 percent of people suffering from insomnia have chronic physical pain.[15]

Just as pain disturbs our sleep, disturbed sleep increases the intensity of pain and the persistence of the underlying conditions causing it. When treatments focus on the insomnia side of this pattern, there is less reduction of pain and insomnia than when treatments focus more on the underlying cause of the pain.[16] While there is a justifiable focus on mood and other mental health factors in addressing insomnia (addressed primarily with cognitive behavioral therapy and medication), the role of pain should be brought more into the discussion (without reflexively addressing it with yet another medication, as is the wont in most sleep medicine).[17]

Fatigue is often a side effect of pain as well as the mental health conditions discussed above, and it is a prominent complaint of cancer patients and those with many other diseases. Although being physically or mentally exhausted might make you sleepy, it is entirely possibly or even likely that you sometimes find yourself utterly fatigued yet unable to fall asleep. This points to the value of resting during the day without napping, as we will explore in the next chapter. When one has chronic fatigue, often arising from an underlying condition such as fibromyalgia or systemic disease, the tendency is to take more naps, which has restorative benefits but also reduces the homeostatic sleep pressure we need for easier sleep onset later at night and for sleep maintenance once asleep.

Timing Issues: Age, Hormones, Chronotypes, Television, Travel, and Shift Work

Although the twin forces of circadian rhythm and homeostatic sleep pressure in healthy people usually result in sleep for around seven to eight hours between 11 p.m. and 7 a.m. (see chapter 1), it does not always work that way. Insomnia still happens, even when free of stress, anxiety, depression, physical pain, and illness. This is often a timing issue, which can arise from the slightly slow 24.2-hour circadian clock discussed earlier, as well as age, hormonal conditions, chronotype (explained below), jet lag, shift work, or something as simple (and complex) as addiction to a late-night television show.

Our sleep-wake patterns vary by age. We might say we "slept like a baby" after a solid night of restorative sleep, but most babies do not sleep all through the night, especially in the first three months of their life, which are characterized by polyphasic sleep (waking frequently) as their circadian clock is not yet developed (it takes a few months for the suprachiasmatic nucleus to become entrained to light and other forces).[18] By age four most children develop a biphasic sleep pattern (taking a long daytime "nap"), and later in childhood come into the monophasic pattern of adults, even as the ratio of NREM and REM is lower (and considered by some to be related to the greater development of neural circuitry in infancy and childhood that goes far in determining one's lifelong capacity for learning).[19] In adolescence we come to yet another sleep-wake pattern—greater deep-sleep intensity, which one might experience trying to awaken one's teenager—within which it appears there are further cognitive refinements in the brain that play a significant role in our healthy development, including our mental health.[20]

Table 2.1. Sleep Needs from Birth to Older Age

AGE	SLEEP NEEDS
Newborns: 0–3 months	14–17 Hours
Infants: 3 months to 1 year	12–15 Hours
Toddlers: 1–3 years	11–14 Hours
Preschoolers: 3–5 years	10–13 Hours
School-Age Children: 5–10 years	9–11 Hours
Adolescents: 11–19 years	8–10 Hours
Adults: 20–60 years	7–9 Hours
Older Adults: 60+ years	7–8 Hours

A related aspect of adolescent sleep-wake patterns that deserves mention is the change in circadian rhythm that makes it natural for teenagers to fall asleep two or three hours later than their parents, while still needing eight to ten hours of sleep.[21] The primary sleep problem experienced by teenagers is their parents' insistence on their going to bed and waking up in keeping with the adult circadian clock, the job clock, and the related school clock. Ideally, teenagers would go to sleep at around 1:30 a.m., wake around 10:30 a.m., and go to school from noon to 6 p.m. Instead, they fall asleep over their algebra or history book at 9 a.m.[22] While other factors that affect sleep can pertain to adolescents (starting with staring into blue-light screens late at night to connect with friends on social media), this factor is common to all adolescents, disturbing their otherwise healthy sleep. (Teenagers rate the highest in sleep efficiency, at 95 percent, getting high doses of deep sleep.)

As we continue aging, especially from middle age to older age, our circadian rhythm gradually shifts in the opposite direction as that found in adolescence, causing us to fall asleep earlier and wake earlier.[23] Our sleep is increasingly fragmented, with sleep efficiency dropping to around 70–80 percent at age eighty, with a weak bladder playing a significant role.[24] This drop occurs even when controlling for most other sleep factors, while exacerbating physical and mental health problems that affect sleep.[25] With regressed circadian rhythm and fragmented sleep, there is a tendency to become sleepy when social pressure and personal interests drive late-evening activity, but accumulated sleep pressure often causes dozing, which then makes it more difficult to get to sleep later. Elderly people who like to exercise upon rising early exacerbate this problem because early-morning bright light exposure pulls their circadian clock further back.[26]

Perimenopause and menopause can be considered a natural feature of hormonal timing across the life cycle. Menopause occurs in women naturally and most commonly at around age fifty as the capacity of the ovaries to generate egg cells that can be fertilized is depleted. Several frequent symptoms found in postmenopausal women are associated with insomnia, including anxiety, depression, hot flashes, and headache.[27] Although hot flashes are one of the strongest factors associated with poor sleep, it is important to note that poor sleep frequently occurs in perimenopause and postmenopause without hot flashes, typically in association with other sleep factors.

Another significant timing factor is that we tend to be "morning types" or "evening types." These tendencies reflect individual differences in circadian rhythm, referred to as chronotypes, that give us relative "morningness" (more energized in the morning) and "eveningness" (more energized in the evening).[28] We can also refer to these as circadian types in which individuals show differences in diurnal rhythms. Melatonin levels drop more rapidly from their wee-hour peak in morning types, whereas body temperature bottoms out at around 4 a.m. for morning types versus 6 a.m. for evening types, and about a half hour earlier for both among women. (Melatonin levels and core body temperature play powerful roles in causing sleep.)

Even though morning types are likely to wake up earlier than evening types, many evening types go to sleep late yet wake up early—and typically tired—to the sound of an alarm, then use caffeine for energy. Many morning types stay up late to watch a television show or to share precious time with their night owl partner, perhaps using caffeine to stay awake, only to wake up early in the morning to the vibrations of their circadian clock slightly sleep deprived as they now join their partner in the morning caffeine ritual.

Jet lag is a timing issue that significantly impacts our circadian rhythm and homeostatic sleep pressure (explained in chapter 1).[29] Our biological clock does not automatically reset as we travel across time zones, and the sleep pressure from adenosine does not automatically reset either. In my personal experience with repetitive travel across eight to ten time zones in recent years, I've found it takes me about one day per time zone to get reset and recover from the effects of disturbed sleep, slightly longer going west to east because I'm moving opposite to earth's rotation, even if the recovery could be superficial. (Some sleep science suggests there is no way to fully make up for lost sleep, i.e., there are some persistent remnants of accumulated sleep deficit effects.)

The timing issues with shift work are perhaps most perilous. Shift work takes place on a schedule outside the common 9–5 workday, with shifts most often ending around 10–11 p.m. or 7–8 a.m. More than 15 percent of wage and salary workers are shift workers.[30] They have less exposure to daylight upon waking and greater exposure to artificial light closer to sleeping, including the sleep inhibiting blue wavelength light from illuminated screens and other LED sources, which directly disturbs their circadian rhythm.[31] They have a higher rate of sleep disturbance and excessive sleepiness when awake, with significant consequences for both workplace and nonworkplace attention, concentration, and motor skills.[32] Think for a moment about airline pilots (especially trans- and intercontinental), truck drivers (especially long-haul), train operators, police officers, and bus drivers who are shift workers. Beyond what you might be thinking about the risk to others from these sleep-disturbed workers, appreciate that they also have higher rates of cardiovascular disease, dementia, and other health problems.[33] Unfortunately, shift workers often choose the quick-fix approach to their sleep and wake problems with drugs, which often worsen their other health issues.

Table 2.2. Shift Workers in the United States by Occupation and Schedule

TOP OCCUPATIONS	SHIFT WORKERS
Production	2,021,000
Transportation and Material Moving	1,900,000
Food Preparation and Serving	1,568,000
Sales and Related Occupations	1,464,000
Office and Administrative Support	1,458,000
Health Care Practice and Technical	1,138,000
Protection Services	1,125,000
Management	612,000
Cleaning and Maintenance	609,000
Personal Care and Support	542,000

TOP OCCUPATIONS	SHIFT WORKERS
Health Care Support	534,000
Installation, Maintenance, and Repair	488,000
Construction and Extraction	256,000
Community and Social Services	237,000
Arts, Entertainment, Media, and Sports	221,000
Total	**14,173,000**

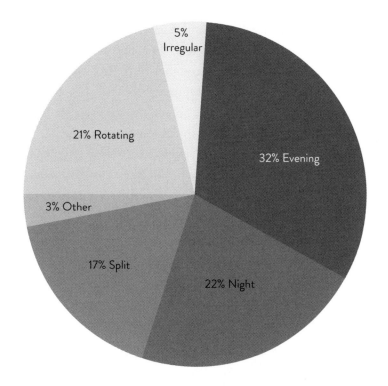

Source: U.S. Department of Labor. 2004. "Economic News Release—Shift Usually Worked: Full-Time Wage and Salary Workers by Selected Characteristics, May 2004." Washington, DC: U.S. Department of Labor, Bureau of Labor Statistics. www.bls.gov /news.release/flex.t04.htm.

Sleep Apnea

If healthy, we ordinarily breathe without thinking about it as the brain gathers data on blood oxygen and carbon dioxide levels and sends signals to our respiratory muscles (the diaphragm, intercostal, and around the larynx) that cause us to breathe. Sleep apnea (literally, "without breath") is marked by periodic pauses in breathing that can last for a few seconds up to a few minutes, causing hypoxia (oxygen deficiency) and hypercapnia (excessive carbon dioxide).[34] One of a vast array of sleep-related breathing disorders, its most common form is obstructive sleep apnea (OSA, which affects about 7 percent of the general population), in which the upper airway is partially or completely obstructed.[35] In contrast, in central sleep apnea (CSA) the brain's central respiratory control center fails to respond to signals of chemoreceptors that send data on blood oxygen–carbon dioxide levels to the brain, causing pauses in breathing of up to thirty seconds. In complex sleep apnea, one has both OSA and CSA. All types of sleep apnea disturb sleep maintenance and can cause several other serious health problems or be fatal.

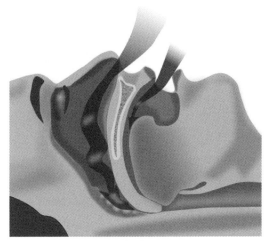

Obstructive Sleep Apnea

OSA and CSA are two to three times more common in men than women and far more common in the elderly than in young people, with obesity a leading risk factor due to lack of muscle tone and the softness of tissues in the throat. An elderly overweight male with atrial fibrillation (the most common type of heart rhythm dysfunction) who is using diuretics is at highest risk of OSA. CSA is also associated with obesity (especially large neck circumference)[36] and the use of opioid medications (in 2017, there were more than 190 million opioid prescriptions dispensed in the United States).[37] (Obesity is a significant risk factor for other sleep disorders, and sleep disorders are highly associated with greater obesity.[38])

Rather than affecting only sleep, OSA puts one at high risk of stroke, arterial disease, heart attack, and hypertension, whereas CSA can contribute to these serious health problems while compounding epileptic seizures, heart arrhythmias and attacks, and the harmful effects of several respiratory medications.[39] OSA also appears to cause abnormalities in several areas of the brain.[40]

Restless Legs Syndrome

With a compelling yet unconscious urge to move the legs, especially in the evening and when at rest, restless legs syndrome (RLS) can disturb sleep onset and maintenance (due to twitching while asleep).[41] It is most common among older adults in the United States, where nearly 10 percent of adults are affected, but is also found in the young. Whether early or late onset (before or after age forty-five), RLS is associated with low iron levels, rheumatoid arthritis, diabetes, and pregnancy, with early onset worsening over time, and it may have a genetic cause.[42] A related condition, called periodic limb movement disorder (PLMD), which involves involuntary limb movement during sleep, exacerbates the sleep issues arising from RLS.

Parasomnias

At first blush, the term "parasomnia" can evoke thoughts of supernatural paranormal experiences such as telepathy and contact with poltergeists, both of which figure prominently in many ancient to modern yoga texts. Parasomnias are indeed abnormal and can seem quite akin to paranormal events. They manifest in many forms, tend to occur in transitional sleep states, either coming in or out of NREM sleep or in or out of REM sleep (but not both), and all are associated with sleep disturbance or fear of sleeping.[43] Some can be entwined with some of the others.[44] Curiously, the transitional sleep states in which they mostly occur are what we describe in yoga as phases of yoga nidra.

In NREM Sleep[45]

Sleepwalking: Far more common among children than adults, somnambulism is perceived by others as though the sleeping person is awake as they sit up in bed and sometimes walk around and even talk, usually incoherently.[46] It is most common in those with anxiety, fatigue, or heavy alcohol use, and those taking medications with psychotic side effects (thus sleeping pills are a prime suspect).

Confusional Arousal: More common in children than adults and similar to somnambulism in that the sleeping person seems awake, in confusional arousal we exhibit unresponsive, disoriented, and confused behavior that can last a few minutes or longer. It is caused by or associated with illness, sleep apnea, sleep deprivation, jet lag, and migraine headaches.

Sleep Terrors: Not to be confused with nightmares (which occur during REM sleep and are usually remembered), sleep terrors (sometimes called night terrors) are extreme night-mares that occur during NREM sleep and leave only vague memories.[47] Although a very small percentage of adults ever have this experience, they are common among those with PTSD.[48]

Sexsomnia: Not to be confused with early-morning sexual awakening of both men and women while still asleep, in sex-somnia one fully engages in sexual acts ranging from fondling to intercourse while fully in NREM sleep.[49] Sexsomnia most often occurs with confusional arousal, occurs among men and women with only slight behavioral differences, and is often associated with sleep apnea, sleep deprivation, and use of alcohol before going to sleep.

Exploding Head Syndrome: Experienced by less than 10 per-cent of people and more often in women than men, exploding head syndrome is characterized by the perception of fright-eningly loud noises during sleep-wake or wake-sleep transi-tions.[50] While this is rarely reported to medical professionals and of unknown cause, various researchers have posited every-thing from stress and anxiety to changes in medication and ear dysfunctions to explain it. There are no known treatments.

In REM Sleep

REM Sleep Behavior Disorder (RBD): Most common among men over age fifty, in RBD we lose our muscle atonia and thus act out our dreams, sometimes violently and with tragic con-sequences.[51] It happens mostly as a side effect of antidepres-sant medication. When not associated with antidepressants, it occurs mostly for unknown reasons or in association with alcohol use or dementia.

Recurrent Isolated Sleep Paralysis: Occurring in the wake-sleep and sleep-wake transitions, sleep paralysis is a relatively common condition (experienced by over 10 percent of people) in which we are aware of being mostly awake yet unable to move or speak, sometimes becoming fearful as we may hear, feel, or see things that are not real.[52] It is mostly associated with stress and sleep deprivation.

Catathrenia: Similar in appearance to obstructive sleep apnea and almost always occurring during REM sleep, in catathrenia we tend to retain our inhalations until exhaling with a deep groaning sound unlike a snoring sound. It appears to be associated with stress, especially in those who tend to hold the breath in as a reaction to stressful events. Yoga might be the perfect remedy.

Narcolepsy

Narcolepsy is characterized by the combination of cataplexy (in which strong emotion or laughter makes you collapse), hallucinations just before falling asleep, sleep paralysis, and attacks of excessive daytime sleepiness that may result in suddenly falling asleep.[53] Strange as this combination of symptoms might seem, narcolepsy is found in about one in two thousand people. Both sleep and wake states are fragmented, with REM brain signals found when fully awake (thus the hallucinations before falling asleep). Sleep attacks can occur at any time, which is why those with unregulated narcolepsy should not drive cars. As this condition is caused by the loss of orexin neurons or orexin receptors, the most yoga offers for narcolepsy is reduction in the hyperarousal that can make prophylactic napping easier (thus reducing sleep attacks), even as doing yoga gives those with narcolepsy the general benefits of yoga.

Stimulants

Caffeine, one of the leading causes of insomnia and problematic for those with other sleep disorders, is the most widely used drug in the world, with habitual use and addiction typically beginning in childhood with caffeinated soft drinks.[54] Over 90 percent of U.S. adults consume it every day. Nicotine, also a stimulant, is still widely used, even as its use is dropping in wealthy countries. Alcohol, a sedative that helps sleep onset but disturbs sleep maintenance, is also widely used.[55] Many prescription drugs cause sleep disorders and psychological disturbance along with a host of other harmful side effects, even as some help with many sleep disorders. Similarly, marijuana, which is powerful and increasingly legal, can help or disturb sleep, and can have both healthy and harmful side effects depending on its strain and the condition of the person using it. Let us look more closely at stimulants.

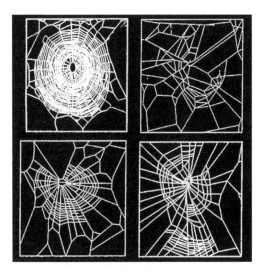

European Garden Spiders on Drugs (Clockwise from upper left: normal (no chemical), caffeine, amphetamine (Benzedrine), cannabis (THC).)

Source: Noever, R., J. Cronise, and R. A. Relwani. 1995. "Using Spider-Web Patterns to Determine Toxicity." NASA Tech Briefs 19 (4): 82.

Caffeine is a powerful and highly addictive stimulant that blocks the hormone adenosine from causing sleep pressure.[56] This can be lifesaving if needing to be alert while your circadian rhythm and homeostatic sleep pressure are making you sleepy.[57] It can also disturb your sleep, especially if consumed in the late afternoon or evening.[58] Along with sleep disturbance, if not used in moderation it can cause or exacerbate anxiety, disturb normal heart rhythm, and raise blood pressure.[59] All of these reactions are modulated by one's genetics and overall health condition. (If you are a coffee drinker with an efficient P450 1A2 liver enzyme, you will be less likely to have sleep disturbance after consuming caffeine, except that as it cleans out the caffeine your energy is likely to drop fast, leading you to consume yet more caffeine, the harmful effects of which are no less harmful for having been efficiently processed in your liver.[60])

Nicotine is a stimulant that interferes with sleep.[61] Despite nicotine helping reduce the risk of development of Parkinson's disease, improving attention and memory in those with mild cognitive impairment, and possibly reducing rumination when depressed, the health consequences of nicotine consumption far outweigh these marginal benefits (and there are healthy alternatives for receiving each of these benefits). If you have insomnia or any other sleep disorder, nicotine will make it worse.

The Yoga View of Sleep Disturbance

Neuroscience, sleep medicine, and medical psychiatry dominate the discussion of sleep and sleep issues. These approaches give us specialized insight into sleep and the biological and physiological basis of sleep issues that can inform more refined and effective treatments for insomnia and other sleep disorders, even as the cornerstones of these treatments are risky medications and a narrow behaviorist approach to sleep called cognitive behavioral therapy (it is very effective), which we will explore in the next chapter. The most common treatments based on these sources focus on reducing symptoms that are conceptualized in narrowly descriptive diagnostic terms, epitomized in the *ICSD* and *DSM-V,* typically filtering out the fuller qualities of someone's life, their relationships with others, and the complexity of their conditions.[62] Reduced to one's symptoms, that is all there is to treat, rather than looking at the underlying conditions and choices that shape an individual's life, including their sleep issues.

The complex nature of human beings and the human condition invites us to widen the net we use in thinking about and relating to sleep, lifestyle, and well-being. In yoga, we consider the interaction of mental, emotional, and physical forces that can cause, can exacerbate, or are associated with most sleep disorders, especially insomnia, incorporating the psychosomatic perspective on embodied memory. We offer this as a complement to, not a replacement for, the medical model that tends to reduce problems to physiology, even as it may obviate some pharmaceutical and behaviorist treatments.

Dukkha, Samskaras, and Kleshas

Ancient to modern yoga is interested in making life better, what is often referred to as liberation (*moksha*) from the forces thought to cause spiritual malaise and thus suffering, or *dukkha.* Dukkha is said to arise from and be mediated by a confused and troubled mind, this as we are living with the accumulated debris or impressions of our lives. These qualities can be relatively latent (*vasanas*) or manifest (*samskaras*), giving us illusions, *maya*, about life and the nature of reality. Caught up as it is in samskaras, the mind does not become quiet upon simple request. (As we will see in chapter 3, samskaras are also caught up in the body, exacerbating sleep issues.)

This condition and the ways to overcome it are the primary focus of the early fourth century CE *Yoga Sūtra of Patañjali*, which begins by defining yoga as *chitta vrtti nirodha*, "to calm the fluctuations of the mind." The underlying idea is that in quieting the mind we come to clear consciousness, dwelling in reality, not illusion. The mental-emotional afflictions or impulses that cause us to suffer, called *kleshas*, anticipate many contemporary descriptions of emotional and mental health issues that cause insomnia:

1. *Avidyā* (not knowing, ignorance): In not grasping the metaphysical nature of reality, we come to identify truth or permanence with the mundane, getting caught up in the minutiae of our daily lives and lacking discernment. Clouded by this confusion, our mind is disturbed.

2. *Asmitā* (self-centered, egoism): The (dualistic) idea here is that when caught up in what are seen as the mundane ruminations of the individual mind, we cut ourselves off from higher consciousness. At its extreme, the *DSM-V* would describe this as narcissistic personality disorder. However, it is important to consider how lack of strong and clear self-concept and self-esteem can cause yet other mental disturbances.

3. *Rāgah* (desire, attachment): Whether desirous of or attached to material possessions or a mission in life, excessive

passion is seen to distort natural functions and lead to addictive thought and behavior.

4. *Dvesah* (aversion, antipathy): Painful, sad, or distressful past experiences and their imprints in the mind lead us to grasp onto or reject new experiences and relationships even when the new experiences and relationships might not in themselves be rationally related to the past experiences, and with the tension in grasping causing further mental disturbance.

5. *Abhinivesah* (fear, insecurity): While fear is a healthy aspect of self-preservation amid physical threat, existential fear that arises from ignorance is irrational and out of proportion to the perceived threat, leading to irrational rumination.

Gunatraya

There is another conceptual yogic prism through which many choose to consider sleep disorders: *gunatraya,* the ancient and archaic (yet potentially useful) idea that there are three universal strands of nature that are present in all things and beings in the world (each quality is a *guna,* "strand"). They are said to give us our energetic disposition, typically unbalanced and thus the cause of energetic imbalances in our lives, including conditions that directly pertain to sleep. First alluded to in the *Chandogya Upanishad* from around the eighth to sixth century BCE, referred to throughout the *Svetāsvatara Upanishad* from around the fifth to fourth century BCE, gunas are first fully developed in the first century BCE *Maitrī Upanishad.*[63]

Table 2.3. *Gunas* and Their Associated Tendencies

- *Tamas:* The strand of darkness, including confusion, fear, despair, sleepiness, laziness, negligence, old age, grief, hunger, thirst, wretchedness, anger, unbelief, lack of knowledge, miserliness, compassionlessness, deludedness, shamelessness, baseness, arrogance, prejudice.

  Tamas reflects a confused state of mind that leads to indecision, lethargy, and inaction. This is the feeling of not knowing what we are feeling or what we want or need. Caught in this tendency, our behavior can become self-destructive or harmful to others. Yet tamas allows us to calm down, relax, or restore our energy through rest and sleep, even as it can make it difficult to rise from sleep and have energy when awake. With healthy tamas, we sleep naturally in the stillness of the night.

- *Rajas:* The strand of passion, including craving, affection, lust, greed, violence, pleasure, hate, secretiveness, envy, desire, unsteadfastness, fickleness, distractedness, rapacity, seeking for gain, favoritism to friends, clinging to possessions, hatred toward sense objects that are disliked, and clinging to those that are liked.

  Rajas involves a sense of intense dynamism, stimulating us to act in the world with excitement and passion, the mind always imbued with anxiety or expectation about how things might turn out. Driven by desire, rajas centers around the feeling of needing or losing something, even to the point of becoming obsessed by it. If we do not act, we fear losing what we feel we need. If successful in attaining whatever is driving our desire, then the mind will return to a balanced state of awareness (or potentially flip into fear of loss). With healthy rajas, we come naturally into the fire of the sunrise.

- *Sattva:* The strand of goodness, light, balance, and essential being.[64] Sattva also describes a calm and clear state of mind, a sense of being complete and fulfilled. Filled with this sense of levity, clarity, and tranquility, we are kinder and more thoughtful toward others and ourselves. We can thereby act in the world with greater ease, because our mental balance is in its natural contentment, without dependence on something external. Sleep is effortless and sublime, dreams sweet and confirming, and we enjoy the sweet light of the day.

It is worth considering how these guna qualities might affect your sleep. Explore using the assessment method given in appendix II for self-reflection on these qualities in your life, one of several tools for *svadyaya,* self-study, offered in this book. You can use it to create a prism through which to gain insight into the issues that make you toss and turn in the night or wake up feeling tired or uninspired for the new day, without paying too much attention to whether it is in the tamas or rajas category.

The Consequences of Poor Sleep

Regardless of how one chooses to think about human nature and the nature of some of our disorders, there are several ways in which sleep disorders lead to other problems—problems that in turn cause more sleep disturbance. In our discussion thus far, we have touched upon a few of the harmful health effects of insomnia and other sleep disorders. There is far more to this story, as poor sleep significantly affects every aspect of our health. Before considering how to sleep better, here is a summary of some of the most common consequences of sleep deprivation and/or disturbance (a significant distinction):

All-Cause Mortality: Sleeping less than seven hours per night or with fragmented sleep increases mortality due to all causes; sleeping longer than nine hours also increases mortality risks.[65] The increased mortality risk from sleep deprivation is most comorbid with hypertension and cardiovascular disease, both of which are exacerbated by poor sleep.[66]

Alzheimer's Disease: There is strong evidence that insufficient sleep quality and quantity is associated with the onset of Alzheimer's disease. For more, please refer to the discussion of this in chapter 1.

Anxiety and Fear: Poor sleep is associated as the cause and consequence of several psychological disorders.[67] We see this in increased reactivity to negative stimuli, difficulty extinguishing fear, and generalized anxiety disorder.

Brain and Cognitive Impact: The sleep-deprived brain is less able to remember new information (primarily due to decreased ability to induce hippocampal-based long-term memory), less able to process and integrate emotions, and less able to cleanse itself of dementia-related plaque in glial cells.[68] These conditions arise primarily from the disturbance of resting-brain connectivity in which the brain's default mode network, its dorsal attention network, and its auditory, motor, and visual networks are diminished. This has profound effects on emotion (see below) and thinking.

Cancer: There is abundant evidence that sleep deprivation increases the risk of developing cancer and disturbs the body's cancer-fighting immune functions. Shift work is highly associated with increased cancer risk.[69]

Cardiovascular Health: Sleep deprivation increases hypertension, causes excessive inflammation and atherosclerosis, negatively affects heart rate volatility, and places you at higher risk of heart attack.[70] These effects extend across all demographic groups, even as there are slight differences by gender.[71]

Depression: There is a complex relationship between sleep deprivation and depression. Whereas insomnia and daytime sleepiness are found to deepen depression, targeted sleep deprivation has shown to help relieve acute depression. As a general practice, sleeping well improves overall health, including mood.[72]

Diabetes and Obesity: The causal relationship between obesity and type 2 diabetes is exacerbated by poor sleep. Poor sleep independently is associated with increased weight gain and obesity among children, young adults, and adults.[73] With increased weight gain and obesity, one is at greater risk of developing prediabetes and diabetes onset.[74]

Emotions and Mood: The diminished resting-brain connectivity noted above compromises our reward and incentive processing and dopamine-based arousal mechanisms and affects behaviors that relate to food intake (and thus obesity and other eating-disorder conditions) and substance abuse and addiction. Consequently, sleep loss triggers negative emotional reactions, making us more irritable, emotionally volatile, anxious, aggressive, and prone to suicidal ideation and suicide attempt.[75]

Immune System: Sleep deprivation inhibits the body from reallocating its energy from wakeful purposes to the restorative processes that are necessary in maintenance of a healthy immune system. Although there are variations among different populations in how the adaptive immune system responds to infection, the general finding is that sleep deprivation undermines our immunities. We see evidence for this with cancer, HIV / AIDS, as well as the common cold, flu, and pneumonia.[76]

Motor Skills and Performance: Our ability to navigate stairs, operate a motor vehicle, throw a ball through a hoop, or thread a needle is compromised by sleep deprivation and circadian rhythm disturbance. We see this in sharp relief among shift workers and elite athletes who frequently travel across multiple time zones for games, and it also appears in more mundane daily activities among children, youth, and adults.[77]

Risky Behavior: The emotion and mood disordering that occurs with sleep deprivation shows up behaviorally in taking greater risks. Put differently, with poor sleep we tend to make poor decisions, including with drug and alcohol intake, eating, gambling (including whether to try to cross the street amid traffic), and other areas of life.[1]

Chapter

3

THE ART AND SCIENCE OF SLEEPING WELL

Sleeping well is all about sleep health.[2] As we have seen, there are many things that come into play in how we sleep, both in what naturally makes us sleep and what can disturb our sleep. Yet for every consequence of poor sleep there are inestimable benefits of good sleep. With our brain nourished, heart in rhythm, emotions attuned, immune system strengthened, metabolism functional, and energy balanced, we simply feel better and we are better. Even with aging and other changes in life, sleep health improves our overall health as we literally sleep ourselves well.

Difficulty with sleep has led to a vast array of proposed sleep solutions, some of which work (sleeping pills, all of which have significant side effects and can be habit-forming) and some of which are modern-day forms of snake oil (there are many, such as Dream Water, the main effect of which is less money in your bank account). There are also several effective ways to sleep better using healthy solutions.

Before making choices in healing your insomnia or other sleep disorder, it is important to understand what is causing the sleep difficulty. Thus, we begin with assessment, offering alternative tools for gaining insight into your specific challenges in sleeping well. We then discuss the leading conventional approaches of sleep medicine to addressing sleep problems: medication and cognitive behavioral therapy. Next, we cover sleep hygiene practices, which have a close affinity with yoga approaches to better sleep and are often offered along with medication and cognitive behavioral therapy. Finally, we look at how yoga—in conjunction with safe and healthy conventional approaches—offers deeper self-assessment tools and a set of interrelated practices for bringing greater balance into our lives and directly improving the quality and quantity of our sleep.

Appreciative Assessment

The first step in sleeping well is to understand why you might not sleep well. Recognizing that sleep is a behavior, we can appreciate that sleeping well is a unique experience shaped by physical, mental, emotional, and environmental conditions, including our personal and social relationships and how our lives are organized around the twenty-four-hour clock. A one-size-fits-all approach to improving sleep makes no sense. Instead, it is important to address what causes *you* to have problems getting healthy sleep.

This involves *appreciative assessment,* whether by a medical or mental health professional, or self-assessment and self-study.[3] By appreciative we wish to highlight inherent wholeness and vitality, even if one is suffering from sleep difficulties or other health challenges. Appreciative self-assessment can address sleep problems and sleep health. In assessing sleep problems and developing a plan for sleep health, one aims to identify the patterns and immediate causes of difficulties with sleep quality and quantity. In assessing sleep health, the conventional aim is to measure several sleep dimensions: "Satisfaction, Alertness, Timing, Efficiency, and Duration (SATED)."[4]

These combined self-assessments begin with keeping a sleep diary in which to record sleep and wake times along with information on the quality of sleep, conditions and activities before sleeping, and other relevant information. Appendix II provides a set of self-assessment forms and queries for these conventional sleep assessments, and yoga-based self-assessment queries to help in gaining a clearer understanding of your larger sleep-related conditions and patterns.

Medicated Sleep

Despite the priority given to cognitive behavioral therapy among sleep medicine professionals, sleep medication remains the default response in both mainstream and alternative medicine, with prescription and nonprescription drugs and herbs taking precedence over medication-free approaches. Medicated sleep is surely as old as the first consumption of alcohol from fermented plants and other plant-based substances. Today there is a vast array of natural and synthesized substances in widespread use as sleep aids. In the United States, nearly 25 percent of adults take sleep medications at some time each year. Most of these medications are habit-forming and harmful to health yet might be considered necessary for sleep under some conditions (especially sleep-related breathing disorders), whereas others might be innocuous yet only mildly effective in aiding sleep.

Alcohol

The sedative effect of alcohol can seem counterintuitive given how after it gets into your brain you feel more lively and sociable. This reaction is from the sedation of your cerebral cortex, where thought processing and consciousness are centered, along with feeling more pleasant as the alcohol increases dopamine levels. The alcohol also goes into your brain's medulla, slowing your breathing, dropping your core body temperature, and making you sleepy. As sleep scientist Matthew Walker puts it, "Alcohol sedates you out of wakefulness, but it does not induce natural sleep."[5] Once alcohol is metabolized after the first few hours of sleep, its sedative effects diminish, causing repeated waking and disturbance of REM sleep.[6] Higher levels of alcohol consumption are associated with worse sleep.[7] We do not recommend using alcohol for sleep.

Cannabis

As of this writing, marijuana, a prescribed drug in thirty-three U.S. states and thirty-two countries, is widely available throughout North America (recreational marijuana use is legal in eleven U.S. states), Europe, Latin America, and much of Asia, with laws changing rapidly. Due to being classified as a Schedule I narcotic in the United States (along with heroin and LSD), there is little scientific research on its direct and interactive effects. There is some evidence that it reduces nausea during chemotherapy, improves appetite in people with HIV/AIDS, reduces chronic pain, alleviates anxiety and depression, and promotes sleep onset and maintenance, even as it does the opposite in some individuals.[8]

There are more than 450 known compounds in *Cannabis,* one of which, tetrahydrocannabinol (THC), is psychoactive. These compounds, including various cannabis terpenoids (essential oils), as well as the major endogenous cannabinoids (such as anandamide and 2-AG), have various and varying relationships with the cannabinoid receptors in our brain. In affecting the central and peripheral nervous systems, the effects can be quite different and nuanced within and across individuals.[9] While the most common effects of THC are euphoria, increased sensory awareness, and altered consciousness, popularly known as being stoned, absorption through CB1 and CB2 receptors can have biphasic effects (depending on dosage) on anxiety, depression, neurogenesis, cognition, and memory. Cannabidiolic acid (CBDA, which converts to the popular CBD, cannabidiol, when heated over time) moderates some of the effects of THC, including anxiety, sedation, and rapid heartbeat.[10]

Different strains of cannabis can have very different effects on sleepiness, wakefulness, and mood. Today there are many hybrid strains of cannabis primarily based on a variety's terpenes, while many varieties blend the cannabis subspecies, *indica* and *sativa.* *Indica* contains approximately 25 percent THC along with a wide array of other psychoactive compounds. *Sativa* contains mostly CBD and only about 1 percent THC. Considering that THC has a greater sedative effect than CBD, it is more likely to promote sleep onset, even if with strong psychoactivity. CBD interacts with a wider range of cannabinoid receptors and thus has broader effects, which are less psychoactive but more physically relaxing.[11]

The effects of both THC and various other phytocannabinoids and terpenoids on sleep and sleep-related factors such as anxiety, depression, and pain seem to vary among different individuals. There is increasing evidence that CBD, from the hemp plant, reduces pain and anxiety, causes sleepiness, and may reduce the side effects of THC; as of 2019 it is legal in the United States.[12] Side effects of cannabis vary widely, from becoming dry-mouthed, dizzy, nauseous, and hungry (referred to as "having the munchies") to having increased heart rate, cardiac arrhythmia, and diminished motor skills. There is concern over its effect on short-term memory and cognitive development in young people, and some people who are frequent users experience loss of motivation and focus in life, whereas others find greater creativity and renewed motivation.

Should you choose to experiment with cannabis to aid your sleep, I recommend doing so starting with very small doses to experience the overall effects on your sleep and your waking life.

Prescription Drugs and Over-the-Counter Sleep Aids

Many prescription drugs are lifesaving, even as those same drugs can have harmful side effects. Stimulation is often a side effect, often leading to yet another prescription drug for sleep. Some prescription sleep medications are highly habit-forming (they have so-called "tolerance" issues) and can have serious side effects on mental health and emotional stability. Meanwhile, medical doctors are often quick to prescribe sleeping pills to patients who complain of insomnia, sometimes along with counseling on sleep hygiene and referral to cognitive behavioral therapy. Approximately 5 percent of adult women and 3.1 percent of adult men in the United States use prescription sleeping pills (more than 13 million adults).[13] All come with clever brand names to make them more appealing.

Zaleplon (a.k.a. Sonata), zolpidem (a.k.a. Ambien), and eszopiclone (a.k.a. Lunesta)—the "Z drugs"—induce sleep (some also improve sleep maintenance). All have significant side effects. Zaleplon is a habit-forming hypnotic drug that depresses the central nervous system and can cause loss of consciousness. Zolpidem is a habit-forming sedative-hypnotic drug that causes dizziness and headaches followed by mental fatigue and poor concentration the following day. Eszopiclone is a strong hypnotic drug that does not increase tolerance but can lead to anxiety, memory loss, and bizarre thoughts.

Several other sleep aids are prescribed for specific sleep disorders, such as temazepam (Restoril) for sleep onset and sleep maintenance (it is highly habit-forming and can cause daytime drowsiness, dizziness, and vomiting), triazolam (Halcion) for those with chronic insomnia (although taken for only three weeks, it can cause dizziness, headache, depression, memory loss, nervousness, irritability, and decreased interest in sex), and estazolam (ProSom) for sleep onset and maintenance with short-term insomnia (with disturbing side effects that include increased anger and aggression).

There are many other prescription sleeping pills and non-prescription sleep medications, including synthetic forms of the hormone melatonin. Melatonin supplements, which come in widely varying concentrations, affect sleep onset but do not generate sleep. Melatonin has few short-term side effects (nausea, next-day fogginess, irritability) but is not recommended for long-term use. Indeed, in several countries it is available only as a prescription medication.

Herbal Sleep Aids

The herbs valerian (*Valeriana officinalis*), chamomile (primarily *Chamaemelum nobile* and *Matricaria chamomilla*), lavender (*Lavandula*), and skullcap (*Scutellaria,* of which there are hundreds of species) have been used since ancient times as sleep aids. They are found separately and in combination with one another (and/or with other herbs) in a wide array of teas, tinctures, and other products. One should use caution with these herbs, especially valerian and skullcap, due to their effects on the central nervous system and interactions with other substances, especially if pregnant.

If you have chronic insomnia or another sleep disorder, especially if with other health problems, sleep medications might be an important part of your well-being, even with their side effects. If you or someone you know is taking prescribed sleep medications to assist with insomnia, sleep disorders, or any other condition, consult your prescribing medical provider before considering any change to your medication. There are several ways to improve sleep with less or no reliance on medication.

Cognitive Behavioral Therapy for Insomnia

Far from the fields of yoga, modern psychology created cognitive behavioral therapy (CBT), a nonpharmacological method of mental health treatment that has proved effective in reducing reliance on medication in treating a variety of psychological problems.[14] Yet its assumptions about the mind and behavior echo those given in classical yoga: the assumed problem is distorted thoughts (yoga's kleshas) and unhelpful behaviors (implied in yoga's *yamas* and *niyamas*). The cognitive side of CBT aims to change beliefs and attitudes, while the behavioral side aims to change dysfunctional behaviors, with each side reinforcing the other.

CBT for insomnia (CBT-I) is the leading nonpharmacological treatment for insomnia and generally recommended in sleep medicine as the first intervention for those with acute or chronic insomnia.[15] Numerous studies have shown its efficacy in improving sleep quality and quantity in several different populations, including those with stress, anxiety, depression, and other psychological difficulties.[16]

The focus on the cognitive side is to:

1. Calm cognitive arousal.

2. Reduce sleep effort.

3. Change unhelpful and dysfunctional beliefs about sleep.

4. Address mental obstacles to adherence to behavioral practices.

On the behavioral side, the focus is on:

1. Increasing sleep drive.

2. Optimizing congruence between circadian rhythm and when one is in bed.

3. Increasing the association between being in bed and sleeping.

4. Reducing the stress and anxiety that can cause physiological arousal.

Changing Your Mind

Our beliefs about sleep, especially when they're in mind when going to bed for sleep, easily interfere with sleep. To the extent that you have insomnia, you probably think about it a lot, especially once in bed, with ideas about how you sleep, how long you sleep, how much sleep you need, whether to nap, how eating and exercising affect your sleep, how lack of sleep is affecting your health or your ability to function the next day, the environment of your bedroom, the condition of your bed and pillow, how your insomnia might be related to other health conditions and to your personal and social relationships, whether to take medications, which medications to take, when to take those medications, the possible fear of sleeping or having nightmares, and … your mind churns on, and on, and on.

The churning mind usually thinks about far more than getting to sleep. Whether it is matters at work, family matters, issues with finances, health, friends, the weather, or what color to paint the kitchen, the mind tends to wander and wonder, the sentences and paragraphs of such rumination punctuated by yet more thoughts about sleep. Whatever the thoughts of the day or moment, there is often a tendency to make them greater or more powerful than they are, generalizing them to every part of life. This increases the feeling of emotional distress, stimulates further negative rumination, and pushes sleep further away. CBT-I attempts to address this cognitive arousal by helping you recognize beliefs and recurrent thought patterns that cause sleep disturbance, especially with sleep onset. This cognitive restructuring starts with sleep education, learning about normal sleep, the effects of substances, circadian rhythms, and how various conditions in our lives such as shift work, depression, and anxiety affect sleep. We learn to identify thoughts and feelings that reverberate in our lives in unhealthy ways, and to identify more flexible and healthy ways to think about and respond to whatever we are thinking about.

Positively Associating Bed and Sleep

Behavioral psychology sees behaviors as responses to certain stimuli, including what you think. Thus, to change a behavior (a "response"), you control whatever stimulates it. If you have insomnia, it is likely you do not associate being in bed with sleeping well. If you habitually spend time in bed ruminating, watching television, or even reading, there is a natural association between being in bed and these wakeful activities (which is not an issue if you do not have insomnia). With stimulus control therapy (SCT), pioneered by Richard Bootzin in the early 1970s, the idea is to control whatever behavior or association stimulates insomnia, giving us these four guidelines:

- *Go to bed only when you are sleepy.* This helps associate bed with sleep and only sleep. (See the sidebar "Sex in Bed?" later in this chapter.) "Sleepy" means you are having difficulty staying awake. If you wait until you are sleepy to get in bed, you are more likely to readily fall asleep. If you are fatigued but not sleepy ("tired but wired"), stay out of bed and do the "Basic Yoga Sleep Sequence" in chapter 4.

- *If you are unable to sleep within twenty minutes at the beginning of the night or upon waking during the night, get out of bed until you are sleepy again.* While out of bed, keep lights dim (or light a candle) and do the "Basic Yoga Sleep Sequence" in chapter 4. If, alternatively, you read, use yellow light, ideally not from an LED source. Do not do anything that is stimulating. If you must eat something, keep it simple, with nothing that is stimulating or difficult to digest. If when back in bed you are not asleep within twenty minutes, do this again.

- *Wake up and get out of bed at the same time every morning, including on weekends or other days when you might not need to get out of bed, and try to get direct early-morning light in your eyes.* Also, try to go to bed at the same time every night. The point is to establish a regular rhythm and thereby strengthen your circadian entrainment that helps you sleep.

- *Minimize napping.* If you do nap, try to do so briefly, for not more than a half hour, in the mid- to late afternoon and in any event no longer than nine hours after waking in the morning. Excessive daytime napping nips at your adenosine buildup, which directly diminishes sleep pressure.

Bedtime

The aim of sleep restriction therapy (SRT) is to change your sleep and wake patterns to increase sleepiness when it is time to get in bed and to increase overall sleep efficiency. "Bedtime" is not only the time you go to bed, but the overall time you are *in* bed, so that you eliminate prolonged awakenings at night. With SRT, in the first week you will restrict the amount of time you are in bed to the average amount of time you have slept per night in the last week (you can use the Sleep Log in appendix II). If you have been in bed from 10:30 p.m. to 7:30 a.m. (nine hours) yet slept on average six hours per night, you will begin SRT with only six hours in bed (perhaps 11:30 p.m. to 5:30 a.m.). (If average sleep time is less than five hours, allot five hours.)

If after one week there is only minimal nighttime awakening, gradually lengthen the time in bed per night by fifteen to thirty minutes for one more week, and proceed in this fashion until achieving a healthy seven to eight hours of efficient sleep. At first this strategy can seem brutal, but most people with insomnia have significantly better quality sleep after this first week, even if still not getting enough sleep.

SCT and SRT stand in contrast to the common method of catching up on sleep on weekends or with power naps, neither of which provide a healthy long-term solution to insomnia. Sleeping in on weekends can feel great but does not repair the damage caused by several nights of poor sleep, whereas napping reduces sleep pressure and can exacerbate insomnia.

CBT-I techniques have proven success in reducing insomnia while also reducing or eliminating reliance on sleep medications (most of which have tolerance issues and significant side effects). Yet despite its potentially widespread benefit, until recently CBT-I has been done mostly under the clinical observation of a sleep medicine professional, thus limiting it to those with a medical diagnosis of insomnia. There are now apps and websites for doing CBT independently, making it more accessible.

Concerns with Cognitive Behavioral Psychology

CBT is predicated on the view that the mind can be treated as a calculating tool that chooses and reinforces behaviors by aligning thoughts with intended outcomes. This might be a source of optimism for anyone who feels bound by their personal history and culture, but behaviorism generally suggests such things are not so important; what matters is reorienting the mind in the direction of healthy behavior. One's psychological problems are seen as the result of faulty thinking or defective cognitive processing, not a problematic personal life history or sociocultural environment. Rather than recommending deep self-study and self-reflection, cognitive therapy assumes it knows what healthy or normal cognitive functioning is and attempts to then change a person's thinking to match that norm. Thus, there is something wrong with the person more than with his or her environment, relationships, and life history.

Even as CBT shows efficacy in addressing irrationality, it can be shallow in assuming that changing one's patterns and pre-dilections—one's samskaras and kleshas—is as easy as adopt-ing a logical mind.[17] CBT's so-called "cognitive distortions" might quite well be perfectly "logical" in response to certain life experiences, so the "logical" process might be less about cognitive restructuring and more about deeper self-study and self-reflection on the path toward greater self-appreciation and self-understanding. Rather than taming the mind, one might look more closely at changing the conditions that give rise to mental or emotional stress and anguish.

CBT-I is the leading nonpharmacological approach to insom-nia, with significant evidence of efficacy, nonharm, and suc-cess in reducing reliance on sleep medications. Some of the yoga practices offered in this book tap into the insights of CBT-I while attempting to weave in a more humanistic perspective that appreciates the whole of one's life.

Sleep Hygiene

There are a variety of choices one can make to sleep better, with even small changes in behavior, environmental conditions, and other sleep-related factors often making a significant improve-ment.[18] In yoga parlance these choices are mostly what we call *saucha* ("purity") practices (explored later in this chapter), or what is conventionally called sleep hygiene. Choices about sleep schedule, sleep environment, food consumption, and exercise all matter, perhaps none so much as choices about consuming alcohol, marijuana, caffeine, and nicotine (see chapter 2 regard-ing caffeine and nicotine; see earlier in this chapter regarding alcohol and marijuana).

Sleep hygiene embraces the five basic points about stimulus control (see above for details):

1. Go to bed only when you are sleepy.

2. If you are unable to sleep within twenty minutes at the beginning of the night or upon waking during the night, get out of bed until you are sleepy again.

3. Wake up and get out of bed at the same time every morning, including on weekends or other days when you might not need to get out of bed.

4. Try to get natural light exposure during the day.

5. Minimize napping.

Creating Healthy Daily Rhythms

Whatever the realities of your life, it is important to do your best to establish and maintain a regular daily rhythm of sleep for seven to eight hours, ideally with a consistent rhythm of sleep and wake periods. This is the first point of healthy sleep hygiene. Getting less causes or is associated with a wide variety of physical, mental, and emotional health problems, and so is getting more than nine hours of sleep (see chapter 2).

Getting enough sleep starts with creating the necessary sleep opportunity, which means dedicated time in bed for sleeping. If your family, work, and other commitments allow you to be in bed for sleeping from around 10:30–11:00 p.m. until 6:30–7:00 a.m., try to make this a consistent daily rhythm. Some devoted yoga students religiously wake at 5:30 a.m. to go to a yoga class at 6:30 a.m. If this is you, enjoy it, and do your best to be in bed for sleeping no later than 9:30 p.m. the night before. (High caffeine consumption is common among yoga students and teachers who, true to their *rajasic* and adrenaline-addicted tendencies, religiously wake for such early classes despite being sleep deprived, caffeine as much a part of their morning ritual as Surya Namaskara.)

This monophasic sleep pattern appears to be the product of modern societies in which rational planning of businesses, schools, and other places is aligned with a twenty-four-hour clock, often in shifts, as we see with law enforcement, hospitals, fire stations, convenience stores, customer service call centers, and many other areas of employment. Historical and anthropological research shows that in prcindustrial societies sleep correlates more closely with natural light, defense against physical threats, and environmental conditions such as heat. The afternoon nap or siesta, a form of biphasic sleep, is the most natural exception to sleeping at night for around seven to eight hours and being awake throughout the day for sixteen to seventeen hours. There are other variations on the common sleep pattern, some natural and others created. Age significantly affects when we most naturally sleep and the length and efficiency of sleep, from infancy through older age. "Morningness" and "eveningness," travel across time zones, shift work, and a variety of physical, mental, and emotional conditions affect our sleep rhythms (we look at how to address these conditions in part II).

While committing to a regular schedule of time in bed, consider your evening and morning activities.

In the evening:

- Try to have your last meal three to four hours before going to bed, and try not to snack within one hour of going to bed.

- Refrain from having bright light exposure within the last two hours before you go to bed.

- Try not to fall asleep anywhere except in bed. Beware of comfy couches close to the television.

- Turn off all LED-lit screens (television, computer monitor, tablet, phone) within one hour of bed. Consider reading with an incandescent light or soft white LED (yellow spectrum), not a bright white LED (blue spectrum, which, like daylight, is highly stimulating).

- Refrain from consuming alcohol within one hour of going to bed.

- Engage in calming activities within the last two hours before going to bed, such as the "Basic Yoga Sleep Sequence" practice in chapter 4. Read your children to sleep, have a calm conversation, listen to calming music, write in your diary or journal, drink a calming tea, or meditate.

In the morning:

- Get out of bed within a few minutes of waking.

- Maximize direct morning light exposure.

- Do a stimulating yoga session. See part II for practices that are appropriate for your conditions.

A Bedroom and Bed for Sleeping Well

Your bedroom is the most important room in your home for health, because there is nothing more important for health than sleep—more important even than diet and exercise. The basic mantra of this sleep hygiene practice is dedicated, dark, cool, quiet, and comfortable. Nearly every popular book and scholarly article on how to improve sleep says the bedroom should be used only for sleep; a few add sex. The main point is about mental association: using the bedroom only for sleep entrains the mind to a sleep mode when in bed. For those with chronic insomnia, even reading or knitting in bed is discouraged, let alone looking at an illuminated screen to watch movies, television, or videos, whether on a large screen or a phone. As noted above, if you must read in bed, use an incandescent light or soft white LED.

Sex in Bed?

There is a vast preponderance of research on sleep and sex, yet almost all of it regards the effects of poor sleep on sex (it is not favorable for any demographic group or health condition). There is little research on the effects of sex on sleep quality and quantity. Preliminary research involving a survey of more than 460 adults aged eighteen to seventy found sex can help in having better sleep.[19] Whereas about 50 percent of respondents reported better sleep following orgasm with masturbation, 64 percent reported better sleep following orgasm with a partner. It is thought that the increase in oxytocin and prolactin and the decrease in cortisol that occur with orgasm cause relaxation. However, it is important to note that the effects of oxytocin and prolactin can vary by context, gender, and individual differences, with one's emotional state, mental condition, and prior experience making a difference in sex being relaxing or stressful.[20] As for whether it is okay to have sex in bed, one imagines that strict CBT-I adherents would object to it during the evening and support it in the morning, as it may cause a stimulating and wakeful association with being in bed. Surprisingly, there does not appear to be any published research on the question.

Creating a Sleep Paradise

To be most conducive to sleep, your bedroom should be as dark as possible, restricting any light from getting to your super-light-sensitive suprachiasmatic nucleus and disturbing the natural nighttime surge of melatonin.[21] If this stokes fear or insecurity, then have a very dim light. Otherwise, use blackout curtains or shades, or if you cannot control exterior light from coming into your bedroom, use a sleep mask. (Sleep masks are available in an array of designs. Choose one that is most comfortable.) If you are concerned about seeing your way to the bathroom in the middle of the night, create a clear pathway before getting in bed and consider installing a motion-detection light switch to turn on a very dim light that illuminates the floor.

The cooler the room, the cooler your body, which is a good thing for inducing sleep.[22] Cooler body temperature is detected by temperature-sensitive cells near the suprachiasmatic nucleus that affect the signaling for melatonin release by the pineal gland. To help reduce your core body temperature, take a tolerably hot bath or shower shortly before getting in bed in a bedroom that is no warmer than sixty-five degrees Fahrenheit. Allow your head, hands, and feet, which are the most effective parts of your body for releasing heat, to remain uncovered. Meanwhile, noise, including from a snoring partner, can easily disturb sleep onset and maintenance.[23] If your sleep is routinely disturbed by a snoring partner, consider wearing earplugs or sleeping in different rooms. Play with using white noise (such as ambient music) to mask sounds you cannot control. Last and supremely important, create a bed that maximizes your comfort.

Here are a few things to consider keeping out of your bedroom (unless medically necessary): all electronic screens (TV, computer monitor, cell phone), visible or audible clocks, wristwatches, electronic body sensors, blue/bright white LED lights, and anyone whose behavior (voluntary or involuntary) disturbs your sleep (including your partner, kids, and pets).

What You Eat—and When

Food is an essential component of sleep hygiene. Just as sleep affects metabolism, metabolism affects sleep.[24] Indeed, poor sleep is associated with metabolic syndrome (MetS), which consists of a clustering of at least three of the five following symptoms: abdominal obesity, low high-density lipoprotein cholesterol levels, high blood pressure, high blood sugar, and elevated triglycerides. It appears to go both ways: MetS is associated with poor sleep (especially when obesity and hypertension are present), with the causal direction unclear and likely mutual.[25] A diet high in sugar and other complex carbohydrates, especially if low in fiber, disturbs sleep.[26] So can eating a large and complex meal. Many foods, drinks, and medications are stimulating. Start by eliminating the obvious ones (caffeine, nicotine) and others that are not medically necessary. Be aware that decaffeinated coffee and tea contain some caffeine. Dark chocolate too, so avoid it in the late afternoon and evening.

On the other side of the sleep/food equation is the effect of sleep on appetite and obesity.[27] Sleep loss affects the hormones that regulate appetite, increasing the hunger-trigger ghrelin while decreasing satiation-signaling leptin. It also increases your endocannabinoids (cannabinoids produced by your body), which, like marijuana, stimulate appetite.[28]

Exercise and Sleeping Well

There is a challenge in studying the relationship between exercise and sleep: those who sleep better exercise more often, and those who exercise more often sleep better. Add the reality that those who exercise regularly are generally healthier than those who do not and it becomes doubly difficult to accurately study how exercise affects sleep. Still, there are many studies that provide insightful findings.

Several surveys show strong associations between exercise and better sleep, especially deep NREM sleep. There is little relationship between exercise and sleep onset when controlling for other variables such as stress and anxiety.[29] A few further nuances are important to note. Timing, intensity, duration, and frequency of exercise matter. Regular daily exercise with moderate intensity is generally best for sleep. Minimal exercise during the week combined with intense exercise on the weekend is associated with higher sleep disturbance.[30] Late-night intense exercise (after 8 p.m.) can be detrimental to sleep because it can raise core body temperature for a couple of hours afterward.[31] Moderate or vigorous exercise between 4 p.m. and 8 p.m. is usually beneficial to sleep. Exercise in the morning, including vigorous exercise, has the best returns for sleep health, although exercise among healthy adolescents late at night improves their sleep.[32] More vigorous exercise is associated more with better sleep maintenance than with better sleep onset, especially among adolescents.

However, if one exercises to the point of physical fatigue, this can cause insomnia, especially if one naps due to being fatigued. If in exercising one creates tension in the body without other exercises to reduce it, this can disturb sleep onset and maintenance. To complete the loop on this, note that better sleep is associated with having more energy for exercise the following day; it is the essential catalyst for a healthy cycle of exercise and sleep health.

The primary "exercises" in this book are yoga postural practices (sequences of *asanas*), breathing techniques (*pranayama*), and meditation. Specific practices are tailored for different sleep issues—hyperarousal, depression, age, timing—as well as one's overall condition (physical, mental, emotional, social, environmental), which informs their timing, tempo, and forms.

Better Sleep with Yoga

In the yoga perspective, the key to health and well-being is homeostatic balance and equanimity (*samatvam*). Although our lives are conditioned by our genetics and accumulated life experience (*samskaras*), we can cultivate balance through the actions (*kriyas*) we take in our daily lives, starting with the sleep hygiene practices described earlier. We can build on and reinforce the benefits of sleep hygiene and elements of CBT-I with simple yoga techniques that can be tailored to have a directly beneficial effect on our sleep.

Increasingly strong evidence—much of it presented in comprehensive texts on yoga therapy—shows the benefit of certain types of yoga in helping to heal a wide array of health conditions, many of which pertain to sleep.[33] There are three primary types of yoga practice in part II of this book in support of better sleep:

1. *Postural:* Postural practices involve bringing the body into various positions that release tension and allow the body to optimally function. Postures can be selected to target specific areas of tension, reducing embodied stress in ways that translate to greater emotional balance and peace of mind.

2. *Breathing:* Conscious breathing is an integral part of postural practice. It also forms the heart of pranayama, which consists of several specific breathing techniques that are relatively calming or stimulating.

3. *Meditation:* Postural and breathing practices invite being mentally present—mindful—in ways that help to settle and clear the mind.[34] Several meditation techniques—breath-focused, yoga nidra (the yoga form of progressive relaxation), counting, and *chakra*-based—expand mindfulness in ways that root out deeply held tension and empower us to embody healthier mental and behavioral patterns.

The Path of the Yoga Sūtra of Patañjali

Self-assessment and a clear understanding of our conditions are an essential part of knowing what actions and practices are most beneficial. This starts by gaining clearer and far deeper self-awareness than we can get from the conventional assessments discussed earlier.

But as the *Yoga Sūtra* points out, we often lack accurate self-understanding (*pramānāmi*), which is mediated by our sensory perception (*pratyaksa*), our ability to think (*anumāna*), and the insights of others who influence us (*āgamāh*), all of which can be accurate or distorted.[35] One aspect of this is how illness, mental lethargy, doubt, haste, apathy, and lack of perseverance disturb us—our breathing, our mind, our body.[36] With refined sensory perception, clear thinking, and informed guidance, we more naturally come into balance.

We can cultivate self-understanding through steady, intense, and brave self-observation of thoughts and behavioral tendencies, the yogi's approach to cognitive behavioral self-therapy.[37] It is a method that involves *abhyasa,* "persevering practice," over a long and uninterrupted period, this while free of attachment to the fruits of this effort (*vairagya,* "nonattachment"). How one fares in this tends to vary based on temperament, whether gentle, tender, and slow (*mrdu*), moderate (*madhya*), or lively, strong, and rapid (*adhimātratvāt*).[38] It also depends on our kleshas, those persistent afflictions that disturb our body, mind, and spirit, clouding our self-awareness.

The *Yoga Sūtra* presents an eight-step practice, *ashtanga* ("eight limb"), to reduce our kleshas and to come into greater balance and equanimity. It is a set of self-transforming practices that give yoga much of its efficacy and its increasingly mass appeal, beginning with a set of practices called *yama* and *niyama* that are squarely aimed at the kleshas. Here we describe each of the eight limbs, offering literal translation, liberal interpretation, and generous embellishment to integrate ashtanga with holistic (rather than dualistic) qualities that can make this path more effective in sleeping well in the modern world.

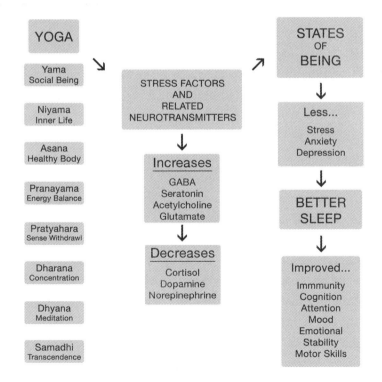

Potential Pathways from Yoga to Better Sleep

1. Yama: Cultivating a Moral Life

The first limb, yama, "to contain," is about creating a moral container such that our choices and actions are honorable. It consists of five principles for how we interact with others, all of which can reflect and reinforce the causes of our sleep issues:

I. *Ahimsa,* to be free of hostility and violence. Hostile thoughts and the perception of hostility near or around us interferes with the calm and light qualities of being that allow us to sleep well.

II. *Satya,* to be truthful. Being honest with ourselves and others makes everything in our lives simpler, clearer, and more authentic. Dishonesty creates complication, confusion, and hubris, which play into the stress and anxiety that disturb sleep.

III. *Asteya,* to be honest in the realm of material things and having probity in our relationships. When honest and with integrity, we do not take what is not ours, and we do not proclaim things about ourselves that are not true. As a result, we are freer of the cognitive dissonance that can pervade and disturb the mind.

IV. *Brahmacharya,* to exercise moderation in one's emotional, sensual, sexual, physical, and mental energy. Through moderation we establish more harmonious relationships in our bodymind (we are more in balance) and with others; when it is time to sleep, we more naturally sleep.

V. *Aparigraha,* noncovetousness such that there is no impatience or worry about what one wishes to have in one's life. Free of greed, we naturally are more patient and at peace with our lives as they are in the moment.

2. Niyama: Caring for Yourself

Rooted in this foundation of moral action, we come to the second limb, niyama, "next to yama," which consists of five qualities that you can directly apply in sleep hygiene and self-guided CBT-I:

I. *Saucha,* the cultivation of purity in body and thought. In taking care of ourselves, in part by ingesting only what is healthy (whether food, medication, conversation, or other things), we develop and maintain better health; and the purity of bodymind we cultivate with saucha allows our spirit to blossom, and with it we find better sleep.

II. *Samtosa* (the complete aphorism is *samtosādanuttamah sukhalābhah*) conveys the idea of gaining happiness through contentment, a quality of psychological well-being that arises from saucha and frees oneself of kleshas.

III. *Tapas,* the self-discipline and austerity that allow us to maintain intense, focused action directed to this path of self-awareness and healthy living. Making changes in our life—regarding food, exercise, work, and everything else that affects our sleep—involves confronting habits that can seem perfectly natural. Letting go of what we do not need while focusing on what is truly important opens us to creating and sustaining new, healthier daily routines.

IV. *Svadyaya,* self-study, whether through self-reflection or study of insightful writings that shed light on one's condition. We are all unique beings, with different ideas, feelings, and even genetics. Getting to know ourselves in any and every way we can generates the self-knowledge that empowers us to take more sensible action in our lives. This applies on multiple levels to matters of sleep,

starting with the sleep-related assessments discussed at
the beginning of this chapter.

V. *Ishvara-pranidhana* (the complete aphorism is *samādhi-
siddhih-īśvara-pranidhānāt*) tells us that the state of clear
awareness and the powers that arise from it come through
devotion to something greater than oneself, a posture of
supreme humility. In appealing to a source or principle
greater than ourselves, we gain the power to more easily
let go of the ego, to more easily and fully concentrate
on what is most important in our life, and to thereby act
with greater devotion to what most guides or inspires us
in life.

3. Asana: Developing Steadiness and Ease

Best known as physical postures that most define yoga today, there
is a growing body of evidence that asana practices—especially
done in conjunction with breathing and meditation practices—
can reduce anxiety, depression, pain, and other conditions that
interfere with sleeping well. Ancient yoga texts say little about
asana, the term typically translated as "posture." All we get from
the *Yoga Sūtra* is *sthira,* meaning "steadiness"; *sukham,* meaning
"ease"; and *asanam,* from the root word *as,* "to sit," which, in the
context of the book's focus on the mind and meditation, suggests being present. Yet there is profound wisdom residing in this
concept of asana, especially when informed by not only ancient
wisdom but everything we have learned since.[39]

In keeping with the *Yoga Sūtra*'s main theme of meditation,
asana was never intended to mean anything beyond sitting
stably and comfortably.[40] So, why go beyond a simple seated
posture in doing asana?

Part of the beauty and benefit of a richly varied yoga asana
practice is that each different posture is as though so many

different windows onto ourselves.[41] Each posture, with its unique requirements for sthira sukham, highlights tension and other sensations in the body and reveals our relative strengths, weaknesses, and imbalances. With experience and mindful practice, we learn to sense how different postures stimulate different emotional and mental reactions; a certain posture done in one way, at a certain time, or in a certain circumstance tends to generate effects that differ from doing it differently or in a different situation. They bring to light what we gravitate toward or resist, what we find frustrating or joyful, and where we are tense or in balance. They are tools for revealing ourselves to ourselves; as such they are also, potentially, much more.

The experiences and insights in asana practice can help us in better understanding and transforming many of the conditions that give rise to poor sleep. Whether we are stressed out, anxious, depressed, fatigued, in pain, or out of sync, appropriate postural sequences in well-designed asana practices can not only address these symptoms, but generate insight into what gives rise to them, helping us to resolve them.[42] Directly significant for better sleep, they can stimulate us or calm us down, help us relax, balance our emotions, and bring us more to a state of equanimity in which sleepiness and awakening happen in the healthiest ways.

4. Pranayama: Awakening and Balancing Energy

The breath is the transformative elixir at the heart of yoga. Whereas *prana,* "life force," is mentioned in ancient yoga texts, the basic yoga breathing technique of *ujjayi pranayama* was first described in the fifteenth-century *Hatha Yoga Pradipika. Ujjayi* means "uplifting"; *pranayama* is from the root words *prana* and both -*yama,* "to contain," and -*ayama,* "to expand." Ujjayi pranayama allows us to cultivate energy in ways that not only contain or regulate it but also expand or liberate it. It allows us to have a nuanced sensitivity to the movement of breath in and out of our body while enhancing our interoception—inner self-perception, which is perhaps the most essential aspect of yoga asana practice.

Breathing happens naturally, involuntarily, and unconsciously. The breath nourishes us and potentially guides us in asana practice and life. Along with food and sleep, it is the source of energetic awakening. Through conscious breathing—using ujjayi pranayama—we more naturally and easily open and sense things physically and emotionally, learning more about ourselves—our tendencies, habits, and self-limitations. But before we get there, we are naturally breathing—or breathing with inhibition.

Natural breathing varies considerably depending on our emotional, mental, and physical condition. Although the average human breath capacity is around five liters, the average actual inhalation is, habitually or symptomatically, around one liter. Our breathing is compromised by many health problems, with stress, depression, anxiety, tight or weak respiratory muscles, distraction, lethargy, flighty energy, and smoking making it worse. Under these conditions, the breath is typically shallow and inefficient, and overrelies on secondary respiratory muscles rather than the diaphragm, which is the primary muscle of respiration.

Yet even when otherwise healthy, the breath tends to fade when we are not aware of it, which happens frequently amid everything else that is happening in life. When this occurs amid yoga asana practice, we tend to lose focus, our attention drifting or leaping away from the here and now. It is more difficult to sense what is happening in our bodymind and to thereby refine what we are doing in sensible ways, thus limiting or disturbing our ability to cultivate and balance stability and ease.

Pranayama practices give us a set of tools for developing and refining our breathing capacity, both quantitatively and qualitatively.

While ujjayi pranayama is essential in asana practice, and while asana practice lends to deeper and more refined breathing and sthira sukham, several other pranayama practices can be done independently of, or in conjunction with, asana, with significant effects on energy, mood, and awareness. These pranayama practices also further prepare us for concentration and contemplation practices.

Transforming Tension with Somatics

The postural practices can be relatively intense. Part of what we are sensing is tension unique to any given posture, whether we experience it as mostly physical pressure, emotion, or mental machination. We typically sense tension as mostly one of those, as if they are somewhat separate. (The word "tension" is from the Latin root *ten-*, "to stretch.") But rather than residing only in the gray-white matter of the brain and somehow separate from the rest of the body, our emotional and mental experience is embodied; the only separation is in how we think, talk, or write about it. Put differently, we are somatic beings, with embodied intelligence that is part of the whole of our being.[43] (This points to the value of the neologism "bodymind"—it is all one. We should stop using "body and mind" and "body-mind" as though they are somehow separate.) Sometimes it is obvious: the stomachache that arises amid acute anxiety, slumped posture when depressed, sudden muscular tweaks in the back when out of sync, physical fatigue when emotionally exhausted. We might well describe such tension as samskaras, psychic adhesions that are in our flesh and bones. With yoga, we have a way to more clearly recognize it, feel it, and let it go.

In bringing cognitive science, somatics, and yoga into conversation, we are gradually developing more accurate and refined maps of embodied experience and, with them, better informed and designed yoga practices for relieving or exorcising deeply held and persistent sources of tension.[44] As we experience the tension that is highlighted by the stretching and stabilizing actions in any given posture, it can invite our more refined attention (or dissociation, especially if we numb it with substances). Placing our attention where we feel tension, we can then breathe as though into the tension. This involves using visualization and overall sensation to direct the sensation or energy of the breath to those places in the body where we most feel the tension created by the posture. In doing so, we discover that we can breathe into the body in conscious ways, thereby more clearly perceiving the tension and more easily relaxing and letting it go.[45]

Doing an array of postures in this mindful way, always accompanied by conscious ujjayi pranayama, the stretching, working, and relaxing of our bodies become a means of working tension out of our bodies, out of our bodymind. Ideally, the postures we do, as well as how and when we do them, is individualized, even as group yoga classes can elevate our focus and motivation. Depending on you—how you are feeling, your overall condition, age, and specific sleep issues—some yoga asanas are indicated and others contraindicated. Some practices are highly stimulating, others deeply calming, still others with other effects, giving us the different practices for different sleep issues presented in part II.

5. Pratyahara: Letting Go of Distractions

Distraction and rumination can easily keep us from sleeping well. Even after we have done our best sleep hygiene practices and created a sleep space that is quiet, cool, and dark, we can still get swept up in what comes to our senses. This is where the yoga practice of pratyahara, which means to relieve oneself of external stimuli, can be helpful.

Recalling the purpose of yoga as liberation from an unstable mind, yoga offers practices for bringing *sthira sukham* to the mind. This revolves around chitta vrtti nirodha, "to still the fluctuations of the mind." But mental fluctuations, rooted in samskaras, evident in the kleshas, and stimulated by everything around us, are exacerbated by bombardment of the mind by everything that comes to it through our senses. Pratyahara allows us to more easily dwell in the mind free of external distractions that otherwise disturb it through sensory overload. Where the mind is hyperreactive to even the slightest stimuli, precluding concentration, pratyahara might be helpful.

Pratyahara can play a central role in sleeping well, as it is one of the keys to deep relaxation. As we explore in chapter 4 with asana, pranayama, and meditation, pratyahara exercises help us in training our senses to be more attuned to inner sensations in ways that bring us to a state of deep ease.[46]

6. Dharana: Focusing Your Mind

With the greater mastery of our senses attained through pratyahara, we are better able to concentrate our mind. As a prelude to a purely contemplative state, dharana, meaning "with concentration," invites us to actively focus our attention on just one thing, even the most mundane activities, from making the bed to chopping vegetables. Dharana practice most sensibly begins simply sitting and focusing on one thing such as watching the breath, repeating a word (mantra) over and over, or gazing at a candle. Making the bed with dharana, we bring mindfulness to each task, from spreading and tucking in the sheets to placing the pillows, present in the experience of making the bed. As we practice this quality of concentration in the simplest of activities, we begin to establish the habit of being present, our mind increasingly entrained to our actions and situations, including the actions of relaxing and letting go late at night that let us slip into sleep. It is also a step into deeper meditation.

7. Dhyana: Opening to a Clear Mind

With a sense of peace in our lives, living in honesty, less attached to things, purer in bodymind, more disciplined in our daily life, with deeper self-understanding, and the ability to dissociate from the sensory world, the concentrated awareness practice of dharana can naturally bring us to *dhyana,* a more purely meditative state in which the effort to concentrate on one thing gives way to contemplative presence. In this cultivated state of mind, beyond memory and reflection yet fully aware, we are just in it, with uninterrupted awareness of whatever is still in our consciousness.[47]

8. Samadhi: The Fruits of Yoga

Amid the fluid experience of awareness from pratyahara to dharana to dhyana, we can get glimpses of something that seems like nothing. Without effort, even the object of our concentration disappears. This is *samadhi,* an undisturbed contemplative state. At peace within and with the universe, at one in the moment, yet still in the fluid experience of awareness, we get glimpses of something that seems like nothing or the whole of it all. Perhaps it is only for a millisecond, as the fluidity of consciousness and the play of the senses and samskaras are nearby, so we keep coming back into the triad of *samyama*—dharana, dhyana, samadhi—in an exquisite dance of increasingly pure absorption in being. We are cultivating ourselves to be as clear and at ease as can be. Better sleep is going to happen.

Koshas: *Mapping the Yoga Path to Better Sleep*

Western medicine typically conceptualizes the human being in biological terms that reduce us to our tissues, while most Western psychology—often entwined with medicine—treats matters of the mind and consciousness using Freud's now-ubiquitous concepts of the conscious, subconscious, and unconscious. The ideas that our tissues matter and there are different qualities or levels of consciousness are also found in ancient yoga, albeit with a very different perspective. In yoga, the human being has interrelated gross, subtle, and causal dimensions, which can be somewhat correlated to conscious, subconscious, and unconscious, respectively. These dimensions are given finer meaning by the concept of *koshas* ("sheaths"), first mentioned in the *Taittiriya Upanishad,* which can help us to map the inner journey of yoga characterized in the *Yoga Sūtra*'s ashtanga path.

Starting on the periphery of the physical body and moving toward the core of our being, we are given five koshas:

1. *Annamaya,* the physical sheath of the gross body (annamaya literally translates as "food sheath," describing that which is fed). In yoga, it is here that we start our practice, exploring the physical body with asana. But this is just the surface. This is a dimension of existence in which we experience matter that is a combination of energy and consciousness, even if we are not yet fully conscious of this interconnection. Yoga starts to happen as we begin to explore and experience the physical body in its manifold connections with the energetic, intellectual, wisdom, and blissful bodies.

2. *Pranamaya,* the energetic sheath, of the subtle dimension. The pranamaya kosha connects the physical body with the other koshas, vitalizing and revealing the unity of bodymind. Composed of prana, the vital life force,

it pervades our entire being, physically manifesting in the constant flow and movement of breath. Part of the subtle body, prana cannot be seen or physically touched as it moves through us and sustains us.

3. *Manomaya,* the "thinking" sheath, of the subtle dimension. The manomaya kosha is composed of *manos* ("mind") and our five sensory faculties, conveying the powers of thought and judgment. Associated with the brain and nervous system and endowed with the ability to differentiate, manomaya kosha is the cause of distinctions such as "I" and "mine" from which it creates freedom (or bondage). Breath mediates the interaction between this sheath and the physical body, which we sense when mental strain compromises breath and wellness, or when the breath leads to a sense of oneness between body-mind and a sense of inner peace.

4. *Vijnanamaya,* the intuitive wisdom sheath, of the subtle dimension. Vijnanamaya means "composed of *vijnana,*" or "wisdom," referring to the reflective and willful aspect of consciousness. Associated with the organs of perception, this sheath gives us our sense of individuality. The reflective aspect of consciousness, vijnanamaya is present to our consciousness when we begin to experience deeper insight into ourselves and the world. Vijnanamaya is still identified with the body, subject to change, and thinking. As the physical and subtle bodies are increasingly experienced as one, there is a deepening insight into the unity of self and nature, ego and the wholeness of the universe. When this experience is shrouded over by memories, manos, the identity is still with the ego, but when fully present in the moment we slip into bliss.

5. *Anandamaya,* the bliss or love sheath, a transcendent state (a quality of samadhi), of the causal dimension. From *ananda,* meaning "bliss," in the Upanishads the anandamaya kosha is known as *karana sharira,* or the "causal body." It is the consciousness that is always there, that always has been and always will be there, even when the mind, senses, and body are sleeping. It manifests itself by catching a reflection of the whole of it all, which is absolute bliss, felt in moments of calm inner peace and tranquility.

Using this typology to conceptualize the nature of being, yoga helps bring the body, breath, mind, wisdom, and spirit (bliss, love) into harmony. Existing as an energetic whole, all aspects of all five sheaths are simultaneously present, interwoven like a tapestry. Using asana, pranayama, and meditation as resources, yoga is a means for becoming consciously aware of this interwoven fabric of existence, connecting the physical and subtle bodies, bringing awareness more and more to a place of blissful being. Along the way, we become more stable, at ease, and fully present to all of life, enabling us to sleep more peacefully and wake more sweetly.

Table 3.1. The Kosha Model and Qualities of Consciousness

KOSHA	LEVEL OF BEING	CONSCIOUSNESS	AWARENESS
Annamaya	Physical	Conscious	Body
Pranamaya	Subtle	Subconscious	Breath, Energy
Manomaya	Subtle	Subconscious	Thought, Emotion
Vijnanamaya	Subtle	Subconscious	Intuitive, Wisdom
Anandamaya	Causal	Unconscious	Undifferentiated/ Blissful

The kosha model offers a useful heuristic device for mapping the yogic journey or describing in the most general ways the experience of moving from gross material experience to a sense of transcendence or bliss. To be clear, the "physical" is never just so, unless without life. Living human beings are always and at once whole bodyminds. Dualistic thinking creates separations, starting with the separation into body and mind. The existence of the bodymind presupposes life, which in human beings involves the "energy" of breath. As stated in the *Chandogya Upanishad,* "no breath, no life." In our awareness as living beings, we also have many qualities of consciousness, including those that arise from memory, reflection, and integrated sensation to give us intuitive feelings and thoughts. The sense of spirit, love, or a power greater than oneself also arises in our organic consciousness as human beings, not somehow separate from the whole of our tissues, breathing, and cognition. It is very easy to lose our sense of this wholeness, especially when thinking about it (or not thinking about it while following someone else's thinking).

Relating this model to doing postural, breathing, and meditation for better sleep, the aim is to recognize where we are in our awareness and experience, thereby practicing in ways that enhance our stability, ease, and sleep. As we have seen, our physical condition, how we breathe, and the condition of our mind most influence how we sleep, conditions that are given highly refined analysis and explanation in scientific medicine and psychology. Going further, the holistic approach of yoga lets us mindfully explore and navigate these conditions, not with refined analysis, but with practical tools that allow refined experience in which we become more whole, healthier, and in balance.

From Theory to Practice

With a better understanding of our sleep patterns and challenges, working with the tools of sleep hygiene, and with less reliance on harmful medications, the ancient practices of yoga can come more fully into play. Asana, pranayama, and meditation help us get to sleep, sleep well, and wake even better.

PART II

Practices

With a variety of age-related, health, and lifestyle factors affecting how we sleep, we need varied approaches to sleeping well. A night owl versus a morning lark, someone with hyperarousal versus emotional depression, or an adolescent versus an older person need different strategies for improving their sleep. In applying yoga practices to specific sleep issues, it is important to align the effects of the practices with the causes of sleep issues. If you are hyperaroused and your mind tends to jump around like the Energizer Bunny on espresso, this suggests a very different set of yoga sequences compared to the practices that help if you are emotionally depleted or depressed, are subject to timing issues, have a breathing disorder, or are frail.

The sleep diary and other self-assessments listed in appendix II can help you identify your conditions, sleep patterns, and which practices are best for you. In each of the yoga sequences given in the following chapters, the practices are designed for specific conditions:

- Chapter 4 is for those with general insomnia.

- Chapter 5 is for those with stress, anxiety, and hyperarousal.
- Chapter 6 is for those with depression and lethargy.
- Chapter 7 is for children and older adults with sleep problems.
- Chapter 8 is for those with breathing-related sleep disorders.
- Chapter 9 is for those with frailty and limited mobility.

In addition to the sequences given here, there are sixty-seven yoga sequences in my 2012 book, *Yoga Sequencing: Designing Transformative Yoga Classes,* for different ages (kids to seniors), abilities (entirely beginning to seriously advanced), interests (in different parts of the body and energetics), conditions (such as stages of ADHD, depression, menstrual disorders, pregnancy, menopause), as well as *doshas* and *chakras.*

Essential Elements of Yoga Practice

The following six qualities are essential in making any yoga sequence more accessible, sustainable, and effective in promoting better sleep.

I. Sthira Sukham Asanam: *Steadiness, Ease, and Presence of Mind*

Yoga is a personal practice, not a comparative or a competitive practice. When moving into a pose, exploring in it, and transitioning out of it, make stability and ease more interesting than intensity and attainment. Similarly, explore all breathing and meditation exercises with an abiding commitment to steadiness and ease in your emotions, mind, and physical sensations.

II. Tapas, Abhyasa, *and* Vairagya: *Discipline, Perseverance, and Nonattachment*

Doing yoga becomes transformative when we show up with the self-discipline—tapas—it takes to practice to the best of our ability. With persevering practice—abhyasa—we commit to staying fully with it. Fully committed to the practice, we are nonetheless unattached—vairagya—to its fruits.

III. Playing the Edge[1]

Moving our body into a pose, we come to feel something being stretched or worked, the "aha." Going farther, we come to a place where we cannot go farther or it hurts, the "uh-uh." We "play the edge" by staying beyond the "aha" but well enough within the "uh-uh," breathing deeply to more sensitively feel what is happening, gradually exploring deeper release. With each inhalation, we back away from the "uh-uh," and with each exhalation we explore going toward it, continuing in this fashion with smaller and more refined movements, and with it a sense of moving into stillness in deeper and deeper forms.

IV. Ujjayi Pranayama: *Uplifting Breathing*

Ujjayi pranayama is the basic yoga breathing technique. This technique facilitates highly refined sensitivity to the breath, which in turn enables us to refine our actions in doing yoga. Breathing only through the nose, with a sense of the breath in the throat and a light whisper-like sound to it, we can better regulate the flow of the breath. It becomes a perfect barometer in doing postural practices. If the breath is strained, it is a sure sign we have slipped away from steadiness and ease. Rather than trying to squeeze the breath into the postures, ideally our practice finds expression in and through the integrity of the breath.

V. Alignment Principles

The functional anatomy of each posture gives us its alignment principles, which tell us how best to position the body in each pose. When the alignment principles of any given posture are embodied in the practice, we find easier access to stability and ease while further ensuring the maximum benefits of the practice.

VI. Energetic Actions

Energetic actions tell us what to actively *do* within the aligned form of a pose. If standing with the arms overhead in a posture called Upward Arms Pose (Urdhva Hastasana), we actively ground down through the legs and feet while stretching the arms and fingertips toward the sky (this pose has more nuanced energetic actions as well). All poses involve energetic actions that bring the posture more alive, reinforce stability and ease, and give the pose greater effect.

Chapter

4

THE BASIC YOGA SLEEP SEQUENCE

Introduction

Even with specific sleep-aggravating issues, poor sleep typically involves commonly disruptive factors, including general tension, arousal, and rumination.[1] Applying the insights of both sleep science and yoga science, the Basic Yoga Sleep Sequence given in this chapter is designed to reduce these factors.[2] As with the specialized practices in later chapters, the Basic Yoga Sleep Sequence includes postures, breathing, and meditation.

Do this practice—and sleep hygiene practices—even if you are doing one of the specialized practices.

The postures, breathing exercises, and meditation practices in the Basic Yoga Sleep Sequence are for anyone with acute insomnia, chronic insomnia, or sleep-related breathing disorders. They will stimulate your parasympathetic nervous system, calm you down, make you sleepy, and help you sleep well. You can do the postures, breathing, and meditation separately or as an integrated practice. The integrated practice can be done in as little as thirty minutes, or you can stretch it to one hour or longer for deeper effect. The postures, breathing exercises, and meditations selected for this practice are done sitting or lying on the floor.

The Parasympathetic Nervous System

In thinking about the nervous system, it makes sense to assume it is the part of us that makes us feel nervous. It does. But part of our nervous system makes us feel calm, relaxed, and sleepy. It is called the parasympathetic nervous system (PNS), with the nickname "rest and digest."

The PNS is part of our autonomic nervous system (ANS), which works through a network of sensory and motor neurons that are connected to our internal organs and automatically regulates most of our physiological processes without our awareness. You might be more familiar with the other side of the ANS, the sympathetic nervous system (SNS), which generates our "fight or flight" responses and often seems to stay in the "on" position in reaction to stress. The SNS tends to get a bad rap, but it is vitally important to our survival and has some sweeter effects, such as accompanying the release of the "tend-and-befriend" hormone oxytocin and allowing us to feel close, playful, and joyful with others.

Whereas the SNS helps us to safely and effectively deal with our external environment (using exteroceptive sensory data), the PNS uses interoception (internal sensations) to help us let go of environmental stimulation and come into complete samtosa, inner contentment. It gives us our resting state, returning us to homeostasis and allowing us to simply feel good. Rather than the PNS occurring only automatically, we can actively do things to stimulate it, which is important in having better sleep (especially sleep onset). The calming breathing techniques, relaxing asanas, and mindful meditation practices given throughout part II draw us away from the stressful activation of the SNS and deliver us into the sleep-friendly activation of the PNS.

When to Do the Basic Yoga Sleep Sequence

- Within two hours of going to bed. The closer to bedtime the better, because doing this practice in the early evening might cause you to go to sleep too early!
- When unable to sleep after twenty minutes in bed (do the shorter recommended times for each posture, breathing exercise, and mindfulness practice).
- If you wake in the middle of the night and do not fall back to sleep within twenty minutes.

What You Will Need

- Two or three blankets folded into a rectangular form about three feet wide by two feet deep
- A large bolster, cushions, or pillows
- One or two yoga blocks (or very thick books)
- A yoga mat or large rug

Doing the Sequence

Step 1: Sitting and Breathing

Getting Situated: Begin by coming into a comfortable cross-legged sitting position. If you are not comfortable in this position, if you are unable to sit up tall, or if your knees are higher than your hips, sit on a bolster, yoga block, or a stack of firmly folded blankets with your ankles and feet still on the floor (it's important to have a firm foundation). If you are still unable to sit comfortably tall, turn to the Chair Yoga Sleep Sequences in chapter 9.

Tuning In: Let your eyes rest lightly closed, or, alternatively, softly focus your gaze on a point nearby. While sitting comfortably tall, bring your awareness to your breathing. At first simply notice it, feel it, be with it. Sense the breath flowing in and out, and with it sense how your body is moving. Notice if you are doing anything that affects how the breath is flowing. With the completion of each inhalation and exhalation, notice the slight pause, a momentary suspension, in the movement of the breath (when filled with breath the pause is called *antara kumbhaka;* when empty of breath it is called *bahya kumbhaka*). Always allow those natural pauses to happen, as they are signs and sources of being more present and calm. Allow the breath to flow as freely and easily as you can for about one to two minutes.

Ujjayi Pranayama: Changing as little as possible in your comfort and the flow of the breath, open your mouth and breathe out as though you are trying to breathe fog onto a glass or mirror. In doing so, sense the breath in your throat and how when it flows over your vocal cords it gives the breath a light whisper-like sound. Maintain this sound and sensation of the breath in your throat as you draw the breath in. Do this for three cycles of breath. Now keep breathing with this sound and sensation but with your mouth closed, using the sensations of the breath to make it smoother and simpler. Breathe with this ujjayi—uplifting—technique when doing any yoga posture, including when transitioning in and out of the postures.

Sama and Visama Vrtti Pranayama: In *sama* and *visama vrtti* breathing, make the pace and duration of the breath equal (sama) or unequal (visama) as it flows (*vrtti*). Start with sama vrtti, with an ujjayi quality. Cultivate the breath by making your breathing as steady and calm, yet as spacious as you can comfortably sustain (sthira sukham pranayama). Whenever doing yoga postures, try to establish sama vrtti with ujjayi as the default. Then, to more deeply relax and release tension, explore stretching the length of each exhalation by a count of one or two, thus breathing with unequal fluctuation (visama vrtti). In stretching the length of the exhalation, do so only so much that the following inhalation does not rush in and such that there is no other disturbance to sthira sukham pranayama.

Breathe in this way for three to five minutes. With each inhalation, enjoy the simple and light ways your body naturally expands. Allow the natural pause that happens when filled with breath. With the breath flowing out, sense the natural ways your body settles, especially as you stretch the length of the exhalations a little more. As this settling happens, allow your body to relax a little more deeply. With every inhalation, feel where you sense tension in your body or your thoughts. With every exhalation, let go.

In preparation for step 2, shake out your legs and point and flex your feet to take tension out of your knees and hips that may have developed while sitting for several minutes. Keep doing ujjayi pranayama with visama vrtti pranayama throughout the next step of this sequence.

Step 2: Basic Postural Sequence for Sleep

Simple Cross-Legged Sitting

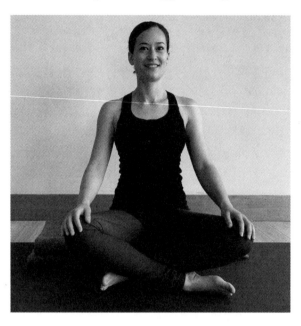

Special Sensitivity: Knees, low back, neck

Props: Small bolster (or a yoga block or folded blankets), large bolster(s)

Doing the Pose: Come back to sitting comfortably tall. In doing so, try to bring your weight more to the front of your sitting bones, then actively press down through your sitting bones (the bones you feel that you are sitting on). If necessary, sit on a prop to get into, and sustain, this position. If you feel pressure in your inner knees, place folded blankets or blocks under them. Sitting upright, slightly lift your shoulders, draw them slightly back, then let your shoulder blades release down your back. Position your head in a way that feels as if it's effortlessly floating on top of your head.

Simple Cross-Legged Forward Fold

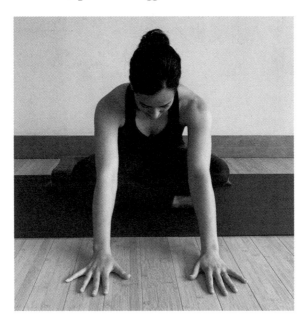

Special Sensitivity: Knees, low back, neck

Props: Small bolster (or a yoga block or folded blankets), large bolster(s)

Doing the Pose: Start by sitting comfortably tall. In doing so, try to actively press down through your sitting bones, and try to rotate your pelvis to where you feel your weight more to the front of your sitting bones. If necessary, sit on a prop the same way you did in step 1 to get into, and sustain, this position. Place the large bolster in front of you. Come back to ujjayi pranayama with visama vrtti pranayama. With each inhalation, consciously extend up taller through your spine. Maintaining that extension while exhaling, slowly release the breath, giving more weight to your sitting bones with the completion of each exhalation. While staying with the connection of breath-to-extension and breath-to-grounding, try to rotate your pelvis forward without rounding your low back, bringing your arms and torso forward over the large bolster(s). Position your torso as far forward as you comfortably can while keeping your sitting bones grounded. Be sensitive to your knees, low back, and neck. With your chest resting on the bolster, drape your arms on the floor and allow your body to simply relax. Explore using the breath for deep relaxation, staying with ujjayi pranayama with visama vrtti pranayama. Let the sound of ujjayi soothe your nerves, and let the elongated exhalations take away tension. Stay in this posture for three to five minutes. Sensitive to your low back, very slowly rise, extend and shake out your legs, and quietly transition to the next posture.

Peaceful Resting Pose

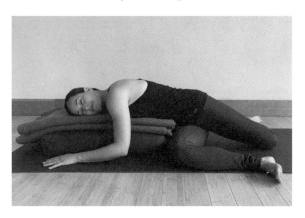

Special Sensitivity: Knees, low back, neck
Props: One or two bolsters (or a stack of folded blankets)
Doing the Pose: Place your bolster(s) and/or blankets on the floor to the right side of your yoga mat. Sit up tall with both legs stretched out in front of you, then bend your knees to slide your feet in about halfway to your hips, with your feet and knees separated about the width of your mat. Keeping your knees bent to about ninety degrees, release both knees to the right while

turning your torso to the right and placing your torso and head on the bolsters. If there is pressure in your low back, sit on higher bolsters. If there is discomfort in your neck, prop up your chest slightly higher and then play with the positioning of your head. (For less tension in your neck, look the same direction your knees are pointed.) Drape your arms on the floor. Staying with ujjayi pranayama with visama vrtti pranayama, allow your body to relax. Let the sound of ujjayi soothe your nerves, and let the elongated exhalations take away tension. Sensitive to your neck, low back, and knees, very slowly rise, extend and shake out your legs, and quietly transition to the other side of this posture. Stay in this posture for three to five minutes on each side.

Child's Pose

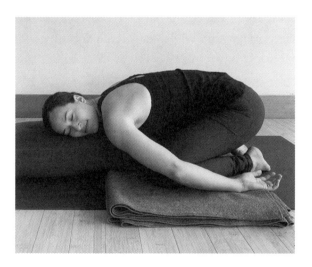

Special Sensitivity: Knees, low back, neck, shins, ankles, feet
Props: Blankets or bolsters, block
Doing the Pose: Come onto your hands and knees (all fours) with a large bolster placed between your knees. Slowly release your hips back toward or to your heels. If this causes tension in your

shins, ankles, or feet, place a folded blanket (or several) under your shins, with your feet dangling off the edge. If you feel tension in your knees or low back, play with bringing your knees wider apart, which allows an easier release through the hips, thereby easing pressure in the lower back and the knees. Also play with elevating your hips onto a block or bolster to reduce pressure in your knees. Sensitive to your low back, bring your torso forward to relax your belly, chest, and head onto the bolster. The bolster should be sufficiently high such that there is no added pressure in your low back. Drape your arms on the floor along the sides of your legs, or, alternatively, bring your arms to the floor overhead. If there is discomfort in your neck, prop up your chest slightly higher and then play with the positioning of your head. Among the most relaxing postures, Child's Pose is a place of rest and inner calm. Stay with ujjayi pranayama with visama vrtti pranayama while completely letting go and relaxing deep inside. Stay in this posture for three to five minutes.

Sunset Pose[3]

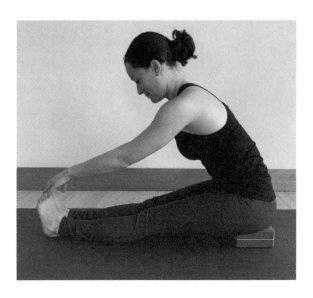

Special Sensitivity: Low back, hamstrings, neck

Props: Blankets or bolsters, block

Doing the Pose: Sit up tall with both legs stretched out in front of you. In doing so, try to actively press down through your sitting bones and try to rotate your pelvis to where you feel your weight more to the front of your sitting bones. If necessary, sit on a prop the same way you did in step 1 to get into, and sustain, this position. Place a large bolster in front of you between your legs (or on them). Try to rotate your pelvis forward (as though bringing your belly up and forward toward your knees) to bring your torso forward to rest over the bolster. Have the bolster sufficiently high such that there is no pressure in your low back, and so that your chest and forehead are fully supported (explore adding a thin cushion or pad to support your head). Stay in this posture for three to five minutes. Very slowly rise, with sensitivity to your low back. Gently twist your spine to the right for about five breaths and then to the left for about five breaths.

Legs Up the Wall Pose[4]

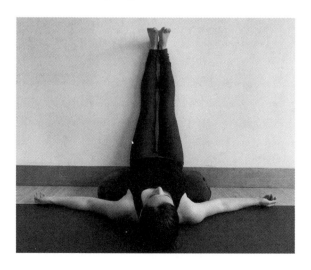

Special Sensitivity: Hamstrings, low back

Props: Bolster or blankets, strap, sandbag

Doing the Pose: Place a bolster or folded blanket next to a wall. Sitting sideways next to the wall, shift your hips up onto the bolster, then slowly recline onto your back while swiveling your hips toward the wall and extending your legs up the wall. If tight hamstrings do not allow your legs to extend up with your buttocks touching the wall, elevate the prop or slide your hips out away from the wall. Let your palms rest on your belly and heart, or drape your arms on the floor, palms turned up. Your legs can be held together with a strap, and a sandbag can be placed on the feet for stability and to reduce tension in your low back. Rest here for five to ten minutes, letting go of tension breath by breath. Stay with ujjayi pranayama with visama vrtti pranayama. To release, first remove the sandbag and strap. Slide your feet down the wall and gently roll to your side, curling up and nurturing yourself there for a moment. Changing as little as possible, either proceed to step 3, settle into a quiet activity such as reading, or slip into bed and fall asleep.

On Meditation

Many people say they cannot meditate because their mind will not stop chattering. Frustrated, they often give up exploring meditation. This mindset expresses the common misunderstanding that meditating means having no thoughts. Although moving into inner stillness is one of the many fruits of meditation practice, it is not the goal of meditation. In fact, there does not have to be a goal. Much like the postural practice, when we go into meditation with a specific goal in mind, such as a perfectly quiet mind, it is frustrating, because even the most experienced meditators have only rare moments of complete inner quiet and stillness. Appreciate that the mind thinks; that's what it does. Enjoy it! If, just as with the postural practice, we practice meditation as a process of self-exploration, self-discovery, and self-transformation—a sense of getting to know our mind—we can experience the joy of it the first moment we try.

In meditating, we open the windows of the mind to clearer consciousness. To the extent that we refine the temple of the physical body through consistent postural practices, it gives us more unwavering support in allowing the windows to naturally open. Similarly, consistent pranayama practices wake us up in a way that creates a stronger inner invitation to the currents of clear awareness, leading to a lighter and more balanced sense of being. Yet to meditate, we do not have to wait for some requisite level of asana or pranayama practice; rather, we can meditate without ever having done a single posture.

In setting up for seated meditation, choose a comfortable sitting position. The most important quality in sitting is comfort; over time, alignment of the spine and general release of tension in the body will lead to greater comfort in sitting for longer periods. With practice, you will eventually be able to sit on top of your sitting bones with a neutral pelvis, which allows your spine to be more easily held naturally tall. For some, this requires sitting in a chair, on a high cushion, or against a wall for back support. Over time and with practice (along with a supportive lifestyle and favorable genetics), you may find you are able to sit comfortably in Lotus Pose (Padmasana), the ultimate posture for sitting (although few Westerners, including those with lifelong meditation practices, can sit in this position for extended periods, perhaps because of having grown up sitting in chairs).

Sitting with whatever props it takes to establish and maintain a neutral pelvis, consciously root down into your sitting bones, feeling how that grounding action allows a taller spine, more open heart center, more natural flow of breath, and a sense of your head floating on top of your spine. Exploring this stable and eventually more sustainable position, feel your spine and the crown of your head extending taller as you feel more grounded through your sitting bones, from there allowing the shoulder blades to release down your back, and your chin to release slightly down. The palms can rest together in your lap or on your knees. Further cues are given for each meditation practice.[5]

Step 3: Mindful Breathing Meditation for Settling Your Mind

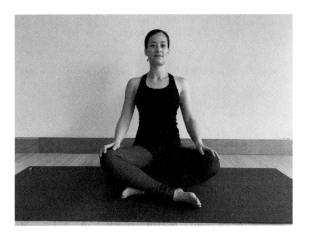

Before beginning this step, please read the sidebar "On Meditation." Then, to begin, sit as comfortably as you can, using whatever props it takes (if necessary, sit in a chair or against a wall). Let your eyes rest lightly closed. Feel your contact with the floor or whatever you are sitting on. Establish more of a sense of grounding your sitting bones, and sit as comfortably tall as you can. Position your head in such a way that feels as if it is effortlessly floating on top of your spine. Let your shoulders relax back and down, away from your neck. Relax your hands into your lap or onto your knees.

Bring your awareness just to the present, to noticing how you are feeling. Notice any tension in your body, in your thoughts, and just acknowledge it to yourself. Free of judgment, simply notice.

Now, bring your awareness to the breath. At first just notice it, feel it. Feel the natural ways your body is moving with the flow of the breath. You might feel it mostly in your belly, in the center of your chest, or at the tip of your nose. Allowing the breath to flow in and out as effortlessly as can be, begin feeling it flowing in and out through your nostrils. Feel it there, and be with it, present just to that sensation.

You may notice various sounds and other sensations. Perhaps you hear a sound from outside the room, or the sensation of the air in the room. Transitory, like the breath, they come and go. Come back to watching the breath, allowing the other sensations to just be there or fade away.

You will notice that your mind is thinking, perhaps wandering around. Let it. Your thoughts, like sounds and the breath, come and go. Let them. Keeping your awareness with the breath, watch it, sensing it flowing in and flowing out. Be with it, present with the breath, present in just this moment.

Staying with it, begin to breathe out a little longer (visama pranayama). Let the inhalation happen as effortlessly, lightly, and naturally as you can. With each exhalation, sense tension draining away from your eyes, the space between your temples as though softening, your mouth relaxing. With each exhalation, let more tension drain away, softening your throat, sensing ease through your neck, your shoulders as relaxed as can be. Breath by breath, watching the breath, sense your body letting go. Allow yourself to feel more connected to the earth and a sense of being invited into a quiet, still mind and deep sleep.

Chapter 5

YOGA SLEEP SEQUENCE FOR HYPERAROUSAL

Introduction to Settling Down

We live in a world in which stress and anxiety are increasingly commonplace. According to the 2017 Stress in America Survey by the American Psychological Association, there are rising stress levels in every generation of adults surveyed (Millennials [18–38 years old], Gen Xers [39–52 years old], Baby Boomers [53–71 years old], and Matures [72 and older]).[1] Although the apparent causes are not surprising—money, work, family responsibilities, relationship issues, and personal health concerns—the means of managing stress are disturbingly stressful themselves, even if not entirely surprising, especially as these behaviors often occur close to bedtime: surfing the internet, eating, and smoking tobacco. Many of these and other short-term solutions are ultimately sources of further stress, anxiety, and insomnia.

Many people turn to medication to help with these conditions, risking the significant side effects discussed in chapters 2 and 3. It is not surprising that many people with stress, anxiety, and insomnia are looking for a more wholesome and sustainable solution through such bodymind awareness practices as are offered by yoga. Indeed, the American Psychological Association study finds that 7 percent of Americans do turn to yoga to reduce stress. The question is this: Are they getting a stress-reducing yoga practice?

In the traditional yogic perspective, the tendency toward anxiety and hyperarousal is symptomatic of an underlying energetic imbalance that reflects a rajasic state. A more nuanced view recognizes that this state varies considerably within and across individuals, in part due to the blend of "state" and "trait" factors.[2] Whereas state anxiety reflects momentary reactions to adverse situations, trait anxiety reflects relatively stable individual personality traits that make us more or less likely to react anxiously to those situations. As a matter of trait, some of us are Energizer Bunnies and some of us are characteristically not. Some people have only a slight reaction to the sound of a car backfiring, whereas for others it triggers hyperarousal, stimulating the fight-or-flight response. Adding to this we find that some people get hyperaroused by choice (watching an action film before going to bed), whereas others get hyperaroused due to stress in their life, including in post-traumatic stress disorder (PTSD). The level of hyperarousal causes various levels of sympathetic nervous system response (fight or flight), including the release of hormones and neurotransmitters that disturb sleep (see the sidebar in chapter 4 for details). Extreme hyperarousal, which is often found with PTSD, is usually treated with a combination of medication and psychological counseling (and where it involves insomnia, CBT-I is usually recommended). Where one has hyperarousal and PTSD, one of the most important considerations for sleeping well is feeling physically and emotionally safe, which we can usefully view as a component of sleep hygiene.[3]

Although doing the deeply calming postures given in chapter 4's "Basic Yoga Sleep Sequence" will help reduce hyperarousal, it is important to go further in rooting out deeply held tension throughout the bodymind. Exercise, an important part of sleep hygiene, is a great way to reduce stress, anxiety, and hyperarousal, although vigorous exercise done late in the evening can make it more difficult to calm down before getting in bed. Although the best time to exercise (relative to sleep issues) is in the morning or afternoon, early evening exercise can help some individuals to release pent-up energy that otherwise causes restlessness when in bed to sleep.

With respect to yoga as exercise, there are very different types of yoga practice, the energetic effects of which can be relatively calming or stimulating. Whether exercising with yoga or in another way, these effects vary by individual in often unpredictable ways that are not always explained very well by either yoga theory (guna imbalance, or Ayurveda's dosha imbalance) or modern science.

As discussed in the sidebar "Transforming Tension with Somatics" in chapter 3, every posture uniquely highlights tension in the bodymind. Tension tends to take hold in some parts of the body more than others. While there are some common patterns across cultures (the neck, shoulders, upper back, and lower back are primary sites for holding tension), there are always individual differences.[4] By more specifically feeling tension in any given posture, we have a better sense of where to focus in doing the internal work to release it. The basic work is in (1) playing the edge by (2) breathing into the tension to better feel it and (3) letting it release as we release the breath.

The Yoga Sleep Sequence for Hyperarousal begins with postures that release tension from specific areas of the body, from the toes to the top of the head and tips of the fingers. There are alternative postures given for each area. To begin, choose those that you can do with relative ease and stability, and over time explore doing those that are more challenging. Doing the postures in step 1 will make the practice in step 2 far more deeply relaxing.

The final posture in the Yoga Sleep Sequence for Hyperarousal, Corpse Pose (Savasana), initiates step 3 of this sequence: yoga nidra (literally, "yoga sleep," introduced in chapter 1). This is a mindful progressive relaxation practice that takes the release of tension more deeply into your tissues, relaxing your muscles, quieting your nerves, and bringing you to a state that is essentially that of NREM stage N1. Consider doing the yoga nidra practice when closer to going to bed.

What You Will Need

- Two or three blankets folded into a rectangular form about three feet wide by two feet deep
- A large bolster, cushions, or pillows
- One or two yoga blocks (or very thick books)
- A yoga mat or large rug

Doing the Sequence

Step 1: Breathing into Relaxation

Nadi Shodhana Pranayama: Alternate Nostril Breathing

This practice is said to harmonize the hemispheres of the brain.

1. Sit comfortably and practice ujjayi pranayama for a few minutes.

2. Place the fingertips on one side of the nose, the thumb on the other side, just below the slight notch about halfway down the side of the nose. Try to place the fingers with even pressure on the left and right sides of the nose, maintaining steady contact while keeping the nostrils fully open.

3. While continuing ujjayi pranayama, play with slightly varying the pressure of the fingers, becoming more sensitive to the effects of the fine finger adjustments.

4. After a complete exhalation, close the right nostril and slowly inhale through the left.

5. At the crest of the inhalation, close the left nostril and slowly exhale through the right.

6. Empty of breath, fully inhale through the right, close the right, and exhale through the left.

7. Continue with this initial form of alternate nostril breathing for up to five minutes, cultivating the smooth and steady flow of the breath while remaining relaxed and calm.

Visama Vrtti Pranayama: Calming Breath

1. Sitting comfortably, start to breathe with an ujjayi quality (described in chapter 4).

2. Cultivate the breath by making your breathing as steady and calm, yet as spacious, as you can comfortably sustain (sthira sukham pranayama).

3. After the completion of each inhalation and exhalation, allow the natural momentary pause that happens in the movement of the breath. That moment of stillness is a sign and source of being relaxed and present in what you are doing.

4. Explore lengthening your exhalation by a count of one or two, creating visama vrtti ("unequal fluctuation"). In stretching the length of the exhalation, do so only so much that the following inhalation does not rush in and such that there is no disturbance to steadiness and ease. Breathe in this way for three to five minutes.

5. Come back to natural breathing and relax.

Step 2: Postural Practice for Hyperarousal

Before starting, review the six essential qualities of yoga practice given in the introduction to part II. Throughout this sequence, do your best to stay with ujjayi pranayama and visama vrtti pranayama. This will help you to bring more refined awareness into your bodymind, to more completely let go, and to more deeply relax.

From the Feet to the Legs

With twenty-six bones that form twenty-five joints, plus twenty muscles and a variety of tendons and ligaments, the foot is complex. This complexity is related to the role of the feet, which is to support the entire body with a dynamic foundation that allows us to stand, walk, run, and have stability and mobility in life. These activities subject our feet to almost constant stress. A great way to take stress out of our feet is to rub and stretch them; better yet, get someone to rub them for you. Here we focus primarily on stretching the feet in ways to remove stress from them.

As our legs transfer our weight down into our feet, they too can develop tension, especially in the calves, knees, and thighs. Active walkers, runners, and athletes—as well as couch potatoes—tend to have more tension in their legs, especially in the hamstrings and knees. These postures will help to remove that tension.

Child's Pose

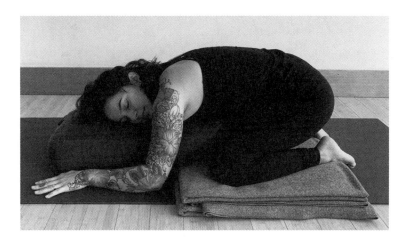

Special Sensitivity: Knees, low back, neck, shins, ankles, feet
Props: Blankets or bolsters, block
Doing the Pose: Come onto your hands and knees (all fours) with a large bolster placed between your knees. Slowly release your hips back toward or to your heels. If this causes tension in your shins, ankles, or feet, place a folded blanket (or several) under your shins, with your feet dangling off the edge. If you feel tension in your knees or low back, play with bringing your knees wider apart, which allows an easier release through the hips, thereby easing pressure in the lower back and the knees. Also play with

elevating your hips onto a block or bolster to reduce pressure in your knees. Sensitive to your low back, bring your torso forward to relax your belly, chest, and head onto the bolster. The bolster should be sufficiently high such that there is no added pressure in your low back. Drape your arms on the floor along the sides of your legs, or, alternatively, bring your arms to the floor overhead. If there is discomfort in your neck, prop up your chest slightly higher and then play with the positioning of your head. Among the most relaxing postures, Child's Pose is a place of rest and inner calm. Stay in this posture for two minutes.

To take tension from the knees after rising from Child's Pose, come to all fours, extend one leg straight back, curl the toes under on the floor, press back through the heel several times, then switch to the other leg.

Toe and Sole Stretch

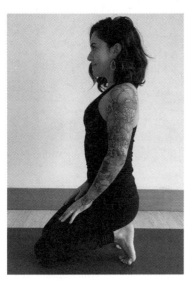

Special Sensitivity: Toes, Achilles tendons, knees

Props: If this posture causes pain in the feet, repeat the stretch described immediately above with the toes curled under on the floor.

Doing the Pose: Starting on all fours, curl your toes under. Staying with ujjayi pranayama and visama vrtti pranayama, sit back onto your heels with your torso upright. Try to stay in this position for one to two minutes. If the intensity of this stretch becomes too much, release it for a few breaths, then try again.

Hero Pose

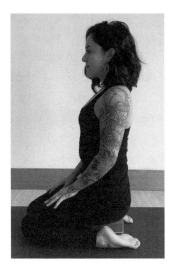

Special Sensitivity: Knees, shins, ankles, feet

Props: Block(s) or bolster, folded blankets

Doing the Pose: On your knees with your feet extended back, press your thumbs into the middle of your calf muscles behind the knees. Slide the thumbs down the middle of the muscles, spreading them out from the center while drawing your sitting bones to the floor between your heels (or onto a block or bolster). Use as many blocks under your sitting bones as it takes to firmly ground your sitting bones and to have no pain in your knees. If the pressure in your feet, ankles, or shins is too much, place a stack of folded blankets under your shins, with your ankles and feet slightly off the edge. Keeping the sitting bones rooted, with each inhalation allow your body to gradually expand. With each exhalation, allow tension to release.

Reclining Hero

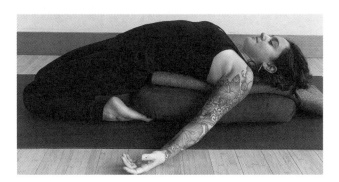

Special Sensitivity: Knees, low back, neck

Props: Blocks, bolsters, blankets, sandbags

Doing the Pose: Reclining Hero is approached from the Hero Pose. Depending on your flexibility, you may need to place a stack of folded blankets or bolsters under your back and head so there is no undue pressure in your low back or neck. You can also place sandbags on top of your knees to help keep them grounded and to increase the stretch of your thigh and groin muscles. From the Hero Pose, (1) place the hands a few inches behind the hips, lift the hips slightly to tuck the tailbone under, then sit back down while lifting and expanding across the chest; (2) recline onto the elbows and repeat the actions in step 1; (3) recline onto the back and repeat the actions in step 1. Stay in this pose for two to three minutes.

Downward Facing Dog

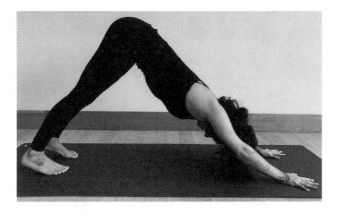

Special Sensitivity: Wrists, shoulders, neck, Achilles tendons, hamstrings

Props: Block(s)

Doing the Pose: This poses stretches and strengthens several parts of the body, mostly through the arms, shoulders, legs, and hips.

Ultimately, it helps to lengthen the spine. From all fours, curl your toes under and try to rotate your pelvis forward (lifting your sitting bones). With firm pressure through your hands (try to press down the knuckles of your forefingers), slowly lift your hips up while gradually straightening your legs. If you have difficulty straightening your legs, play with a wider foot stance; it is okay to keep your knees bent, too. When you first come into the pose, play with bicycling your legs and twisting through your torso, thereby more easily feeling into the pose by releasing initial tension. Pressing through your hands, try to roll your shoulder blades out away from your spine. If it is okay with your neck, align your ears with your arms so your neck is in its natural form; otherwise, support your forehead with a block. Firm your thighs and press the tops of your thighs back to lengthen your spine. Start with holding this pose for a few breaths, rest on all fours for a few breaths, then come into it again, gradually holding for up to two minutes. Rest on all fours or in Child's Pose.

Low Lunge

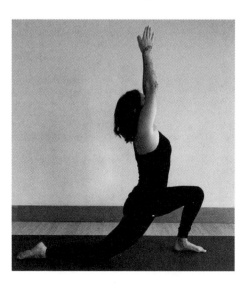

Special Sensitivity: Knees, groin, low back

Props: Additional padding under the knee that's on the floor

Doing the Pose: From all fours, step the right foot back, releasing that knee to the floor, then come to an upright position through your upper body. If the pressure of your knee on the floor is too much, pad it. With your hands on your hips, partially straighten the front leg, and place your hands on your hips to get them level while lengthening your tailbone toward the floor. Slowly bend your front knee to deepen the lunge, using your hands on your hips to keep your pelvis and torso upright. Play with slowly moving in and out of the full depth of the lunge, gradually releasing into a deeper stretch in the hips and groin. Going further, play with reaching your arms out and up overhead. The arms can be held shoulder-distance apart, or if you can keep your elbows straight, try to press your palms together overhead while lifting through your sides, chest, back, arms, and fingertips. Try to hold for one to two minutes, then switch sides.

Wide-Angle Forward Fold

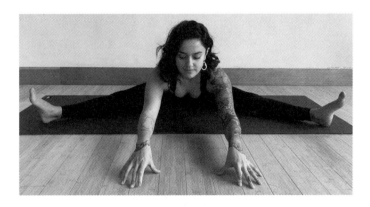

Special Sensitivity: Hamstrings, inner thighs, low back

Props: Blocks, bolster, folded blanket

Doing the Pose: From a simple seated position, separate your legs into a V shape, as wide as is comfortable. If you tend to slump in your low back—even a little—sit on a prop. Point your toes and kneecaps straight up while firming your thighs, elongating your spine, and expanding across your chest. Press the hands into the floor behind the hips to help rotate your pelvis forward. If you are able to sit tall on your sitting bones with your hands off the floor, reach your arms forward and use your hands on the floor to help draw your torso forward. Keeping your sitting bones rooted, legs active, and kneecaps pointing up, move with the breath to fold forward through the rotation of your pelvis, eventually bringing the chest to the floor and clasping the feet or resting your chest and forehead on props. Be more interested in a long spine and open heart than folding down. Hold for two to three minutes.

Knees to Chest

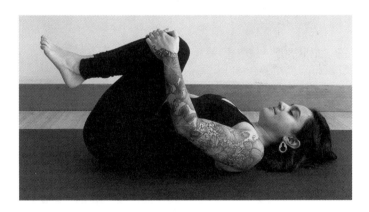

Special Sensitivity: Knees and low back
Props: None
Doing the Pose: Lying on your back, slide your feet in toward your hips, then clasp your knees to draw them in toward your chest.

With each inhalation, release your knees away from your chest. With each exhalation, draw them in a little closer. If you feel pressure in your knees, clasp behind them so they do not fully bend. Play with this movement for one to two minutes, releasing tension around your upper legs and hips, and in your low back.

Reclined Hamstring Stretch

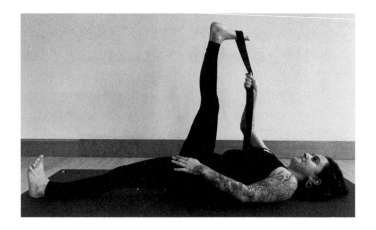

Special Sensitivity: Hamstrings

Props: Strap

Doing the Pose: Lying supine with your feet on the floor near your hips, clasp your right foot and straighten your right leg up toward the ceiling while keeping your right shoulder on the floor (if necessary, use a strap around your foot). Explore gradually straightening your left leg out onto the floor, pressing out through the heel while keeping the knee and toes pointing up. With each inhalation, bend your right knee just enough to eliminate any strong stretching sensation in the back of your leg and around the knee. With each exhalation, slowly press your right leg straight. Maintaining dynamic tension through the strap, continue this movement for one minute, then hold at the point of maximum comfortable stretch for one more minute. Switch sides.

The Hips and Pelvis

Mediating between the upper body and the legs, the pelvis is the hub of the body. Cradled within we find our lower abdominal organs and, in the view of tantric yoga, the resting place of the *kundalini shakti* energy. It can also be a not so restful place where deeply held emotional tension, especially fear and anger, is said to reside. It is a primary center of stability and ease, where we both originate key movements and cushion the impact of those movements through the bones, muscles, ligaments, and energetic actions emanating from within and around this vital structure, including the hip joints on the sides of the pelvis. Because the pelvis is a strong, stabilizing structure, pelvic postural imbalances, traumas, and injuries tend to manifest below in the knees or above in the spine and upper body, while wear and tear in the hip alone can cause debilitating pain that in some cases finds relief only through replacement of the joint. With about thirty muscles giving support to hip movement and stability, there is much here to work with in releasing tension.

Cobbler

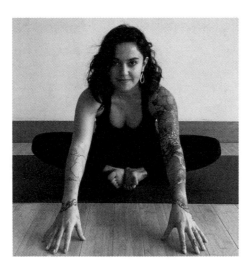

Special Sensitivity: Knees, low back, inner thighs

Props: Blocks, bolsters, blankets

Doing the Pose: From the preparatory position for the Wide-Angle Forward Fold described earlier, bend your knees to bring the feet together while releasing the knees apart toward the floor. If you tend to slump in your low back—even a little—sit on a prop. Reduce knee strain by placing a block under your knees. Press the hands onto the floor behind your hips to help rotate your pelvis forward. If able to sit tall on your sitting bones with your hands off the floor, clasp and open the soles of your feet like a book, pressing your heels together while releasing your knees out toward the floor. Try to rotate your pelvis forward to draw your chest toward the horizon. Next, reach your hands forward onto the floor to help to lift and elongate your spine, and to more deeply stretch your hips. Keeping your sitting bones rooted, heels pressed together, shoulder blades down your back, and collarbones spread apart, rest your chest and forehead on a stack of bolsters. Stay for two to three minutes.

Thread the Needle

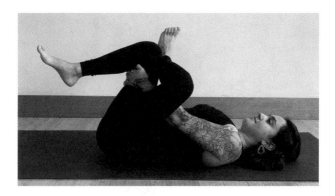

Special Sensitivity: Knees, low back, neck

Props: Block, wall

Doing the Pose: Lying supine with your feet on the floor near your hips, cross your left ankle onto your right knee, flexing the ankle to protect your left knee. Clasp your hands behind your right knee and gently pull your right knee in as though toward your right shoulder. If unable to cross your ankle to the knee or to easily clasp behind your knee, elevate your right foot onto a block about a foot forward from your right hip, or, alternatively, place your right foot on a wall, then cross your left ankle onto the right knee. If in clasping, your shoulders lift off the floor, causing an arch in your neck, use the foot-on-block form. Otherwise, keeping your tailbone on the floor, with each inhalation release your right knee away from your right shoulder, and with each exhalation draw it toward that shoulder (without letting your tailbone lift). Continue this movement for one minute, then hold for one minute. Switch sides.

<h3 style="text-align:center">Reclined Inner Hip Stretch</h3>

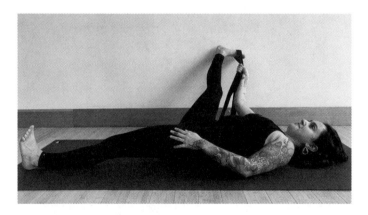

Special Sensitivity: Inner thigh, low back
Props: Strap, bolster or block
Doing the Pose: Begin as for the Reclined Hamstring Stretch pose described above with a strap looped around your right foot

and your left leg extended straight forward on the floor. Press your left hand firmly down on top of your left thigh, helping to ground your left hip to the floor. Slowly stretch your right leg over to the right, going only so far as you can without letting your left hip lift. If the stretch in your left leg is too intense, place a block or bolster under it. Hold for two to three minutes. After switching sides, place both feet on the floor near your hips and let your knees rest together for several relaxing breaths.

Reclined Outer Thigh Stretch

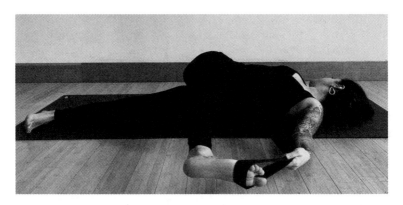

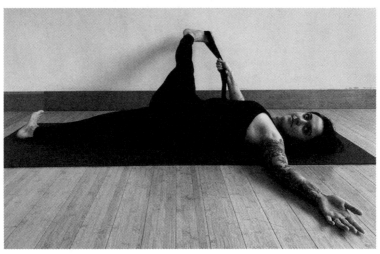

Special Sensitivity: Low back, knees (especially when stretching the IT band)

Props: Blocks, strap

Doing the Pose: Lying supine with your knees in toward your chest, stretch your left leg straight out onto the floor. Draw your right knee across your body to come into a twist through your torso. If you have low back issues or feel tension in your low back, place a block between your knees and/or under the lower knee before twisting. Be more interested in keeping your shoulders on the floor than getting the knee to the floor. With the upper leg straight, place a strap around the foot to help draw the leg farther across, bringing a deep stretch to the outside of your hip and iliotibial (IT) band. Hold for two to three minutes. Switch sides.

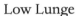

Low Lunge

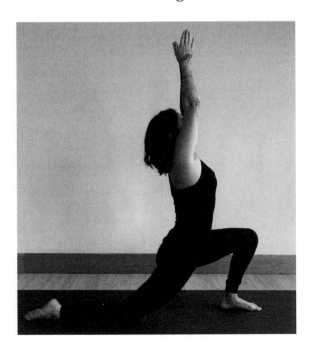

Special Sensitivity: Knees, groin, low back

Props: Additional padding under the knee that's on the floor

Doing the Pose: From all fours, step the right foot back, releasing that knee to the floor, then come to an upright position through your upper body. If the pressure of your knee on the floor is too much, pad it. With your hands on your hips, partially straighten the front leg, and place your hands on your hips to get the hips level while lengthening your tailbone toward the floor. Slowly bend your front knee to deepen the lunge, using your hands on your hips to keep your pelvis and torso upright. Play with slowly moving in and out of the full depth of the lunge, gradually releasing into a deeper stretch in the hips and groin. Going further, play with reaching your arms out and up overhead. The arms can be held shoulder-distance apart, or if you can keep your elbows straight, try to press your palms together overhead while lifting through your sides, chest, back, arms, and fingertips. Try to hold for one to two minutes, then switch sides.

Cow Face Pose

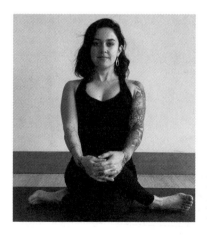 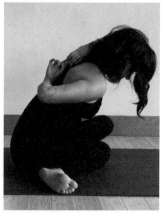

Special Sensitivity: Knees, low back, shoulders

Props: Block or bolster, strap

Doing the Pose: Starting on all fours, cross your left knee behind and across your right knee to the floor; have a block waiting under your sitting bones before sitting down. With your right knee on top, reach your left arm overhead, bending the elbow to draw the hand down your back while drawing your right arm around behind your back and reaching up to clasp the left fingers (use a strap if needed). As an alternative to this arm position, clasp your upper knee with your hands to help elongate your spine, or, if folding forward, place your hands on the floor. Rooting the sitting bones, inhaling, lift your spine and chest; exhaling, fold forward. As with all seated forward bends, keep your sitting bones grounded while lengthening your spine and folding forward. As an alternative, stay with Thread the Needle (described above). Hold for two minutes, then stretch out your legs on the way to the other side.

Resting Cobbler

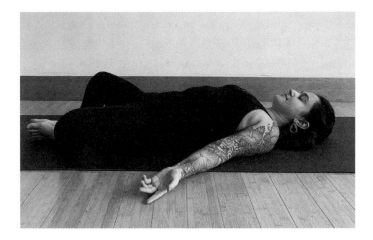

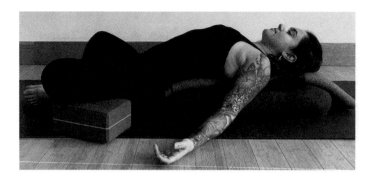

Special Sensitivity: Knees, inner thighs, low back
Props: Block, bolsters, folded blankets, sandbags
Doing the Pose: Set up for Cobbler as described earlier, with folded blankets or bolsters stacked behind you. Slowly recline back with your hands on the floor behind you, easing your back and head onto the blankets or bolsters. Place blocks under your knees if there is intense pressure in the inner knees or thighs. If you want a deeper stretch, place sandbags on your knees.

The Spine and Torso

The spine, centered in the torso, is at the center of life. In ancient yoga texts we find it as the *sushumna* channel, carrying life-force *kundalini shakti* energy up through the subtle body. Its relative stability, mobility, and overall functioning (or dysfunctioning, along with associated pain) are among the primary motivations people have for doing yoga. More than any other part of the skeleton, the spine is directly involved in nearly everything we do. With a greater and more stable range of motion in the spine and throughout the torso, we experience more ease and sensory awakening throughout the entire bodymind. When the spine is unbalanced due to over-developed or weak muscles, repetitive stress, organic tension, or emotional gripping, we see a variety of problems: shallow breathing, back pain, and many health issues; it also makes sitting in meditation unnecessarily difficult.

Knees to Chest

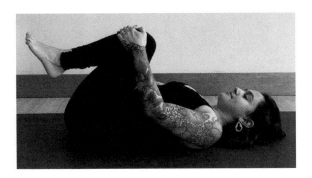

Special Sensitivity: Knees and low back

Props: None

Doing the Pose: Lying on your back, slide your feet in toward your hips, then clasp your knees to draw them in toward your chest. With each inhalation, release your knees away from your chest. With each exhalation, draw them in a little closer. If you feel pressure in your knees, clasp behind them so they do not fully bend. Play with this movement for one to two minutes, releasing tension around your upper legs and hips, and in your low back.

Supine Twist

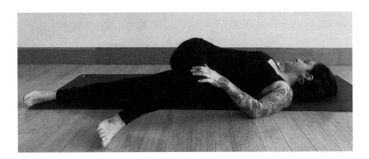

Special Sensitivity: Low back, knees

Props: Blocks

Doing the Pose: Lying supine with your knees in toward your chest, stretch your left leg straight out onto the floor. Draw your right knee across your body to come into a twist through your torso. If you have low back issues or feel tension in your low back, keep your knees bent and place a block between your knees and/or under the lower knee before twisting. Be more interested in keeping your shoulders on the floor than getting the knee to the floor. Switch sides.

Peaceful Resting

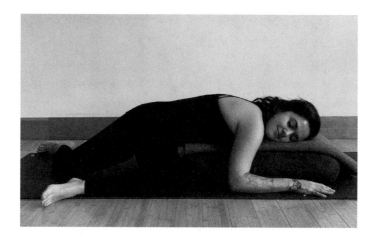

Special Sensitivity: Knees, low back, neck

Props: One or two bolsters (or a stack of folded blankets)

Doing the Pose: Place your bolster(s) and/or blankets on the floor to the left side of your yoga mat. Sit up tall with both legs stretched out in front of you, then bend your knees to slide your feet in about halfway to your hips, with your feet and knees separated about the width of your mat. Keeping your knees bent to about ninety degrees, release both knees to the left while turning your torso to the left and placing your torso and head on the bolsters. If there is pressure in your low back, sit on higher bolsters. If there is discomfort in your neck, prop up your chest slightly higher and then play with the positioning of your head. (For less tension in your neck, look the same direction your knees are pointed.) Drape your arms on the floor. Staying with ujjayi pranayama with visama vrtti pranayama, allow your body to relax. Let the sound of ujjayi soothe your nerves, and let the elongated exhalations take away tension. Sensitive to your neck, low back, and knees, very slowly rise, extend and shake out your legs, and quietly transition to the other side of this posture. Stay in this posture for three to five minutes on each side.

Bridge

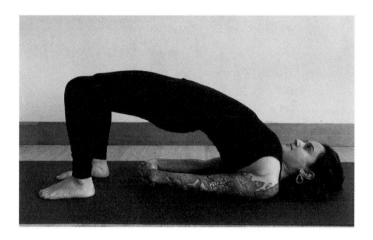

Special Sensitivity: Neck, knees, low back
Props: Blankets, block
Doing the Pose: Lying supine, slide the feet in close to the buttocks, hip-distance apart and parallel. If you have neck issues, lie with your back and shoulders elevated on folded blankets, your head on the floor. Consider placing a block between your thighs

to help align your legs. With completion of the exhalation, feel the lower back press toward the floor and the tailbone curl up. With the inhalation, press through the feet (strong *pada bandha*) to lift the hips up with a feeling of the inner thighs spiraling down, the tailbone leading the way, to keep space in the lower back. Interlace the fingers under the back and shrug the shoulders slightly under, just enough to draw any pressure off the neck. Maintaining pada bandha and the internal rotation of the femurs, press down more firmly through the feet to lift the hips. Pressing down through the shoulders, elbows, and wrists, press the tips of the shoulder blades in toward the heart while lifting the sternum toward the chin and spreading broadly across the upper back and collarbones. To release, lift the heels, reach the arms overhead, and slowly roll down one vertebra at a time.

Sage

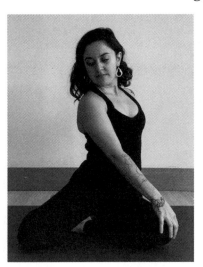

Special Sensitivity: Knees, low back, neck

Props: Blocks, bolster or folded blankets

Doing the Pose: Sitting on your heels as you would in preparing for Child's Pose, slide off your heels to the left and separate your knees wide apart. If there is tension in your knees or you are unable to sit up with no slouching in your low back, sit on a block or firm bolster. Place your left hand on the floor next to your left hip (or on a block if you are unable to easily press your hand into the floor while maintaining a tall spine). Turning your torso to the left, either keep your left hand on the block or reach the left hand around behind your back to clasp a piece of clothing near your right hip or the right inner thigh. Clasp your left knee with your right hand. Rooting your sitting bones, elongate your spine with each inhalation, then use the hand clasps to leverage the twist with each exhalation. Create a feeling of drawing your upper spine in toward your chest while drawing your shoulder blades down your back and spreading your collarbones. While twisting your torso to the left, turn your head to the right, drawing your chin slightly down toward the right shoulder (being sensitive to your neck). Switch sides.

Sunset

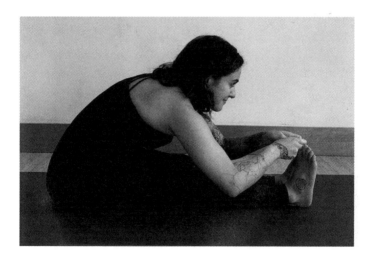

Special Sensitivity: Low back, hamstrings, neck
Props: Blankets or bolsters, block
Doing the Pose: Sit up tall with both legs stretched out in front of you. In doing so, try to actively press down through your sitting bones and try to rotate your pelvis to where you feel your weight more to the front of your sitting bones. If necessary, sit

on a prop the same way you did in step 1 to get into, and sustain, this position. Place a large bolster in front of you between your legs (or on them). Try to rotate your pelvis forward (as though bringing your belly up and forward toward your knees) to bring your torso forward to rest over the bolster. Have the bolster sufficiently high such that there is no pressure in your low back, and so that your chest and forehead are fully supported (explore adding a thin cushion or pad to support your head). Stay in this posture for two to three minutes. Very slowly rise, with sensitivity to your low back.

The Arms and Shoulders

Much of human life and consciousness is predicated not just on our ability to erect elaborate structures or actions in our complex minds, but also on our ability to fashion those ideas into material reality in the world. In this creative expression, we largely depend on the manipulative abilities of our arms and hands, the relatively free movement of which rests on the mobility of our shoulders. Although our shoulder joints are the most mobile joints in the human body, they must also be strong enough to allow us to lift, push, pull, twist, and move with or against force in multiple directions. Indeed, human consciousness itself and the very fabric of human thought are inextricably intertwined with this uniquely human ability to engage creatively with the physical world in often fine and elaborate ways allowed by the shoulders, arms, and hands. The humble shoulders, where we carry much of our responsibility, or sometimes a chip (and where the Hindu god Shiva carries a resting cobra), determine much about our posture and movement in the world. Given the considerable mobility of the shoulder, these precious tools are among the most vulnerable parts of the human body. Take it easy with these postures.

Eagle Arms

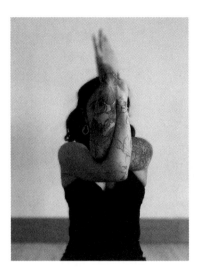

Special Sensitivity: Arms, wrists, shoulders, neck
Props: None
Doing the Pose: Sitting or standing, reach your arms out level with your shoulders, then draw them forward, crossing your left arm over your right arm. If possible, rotate your forearms to point up and try to bring your palms together or press your right fingertips into the base of your left thumb. If unable to fully cross the elbows or rotate your forearms to point up, use your right arm to pull your left arm across your chest. Draw your shoulder blades down away from your neck and against the back ribs. Try to keep your elbows at shoulder height, squeeze your elbows into each other (if they are together), press your hands away from your face, stay tall through your spine, and breathe deeply. Hold this position while breathing deeply and exploring very slight movements of the head in every direction except back. Do not hyperextend the neck. Explore for two minutes, then switch sides.

Front Shoulder Stretch

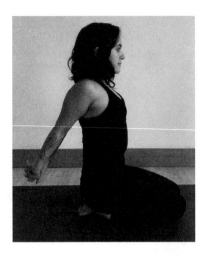

Special Sensitivity: Front of your shoulders

Props: Strap

Doing the Pose: Standing or sitting comfortably tall, interlace your fingers behind your back. If this is difficult or impossible, causes strain in your shoulders, or causes your chest to even slightly collapse, use a strap between your hands, clasping it with your arms shoulder-distance apart or wider. With each inhalation, lift your chest while bringing your hands toward the backs of your hips while pulling your shoulder blades down your back. With each exhalation, try to maintain the space across your chest while lifting your arms away from your back. Do this ten to fifteen times before holding your arms up and back for one minute.

Melting Heart Pose

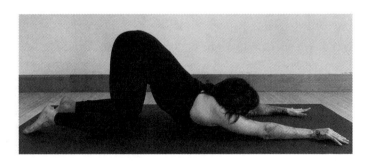

Special Sensitivity: Neck, shoulders
Props: Block or blanket

Doing the Pose: Begin on all fours. Reach your arms forward on the floor and press your hands and fingers firmly and evenly down. Try to rotate your shoulder blades out away from your spine. With each inhalation, lift your chest up away from the floor. With each exhalation, stretch your chest toward the floor. Repeat ten to fifteen times before holding your chest toward the floor for up to two minutes.

The Hands and Wrists

Human evolution is largely due to our ability to hold and manipulate objects, an ability crucially afforded by our opposable thumb. In yoga, the hand provides one of the most important foundational anchors, included in all the arm balances, many backbends, even leveraged hip openers, twists, and forward bends. Given considerable mobility by the wrist joint, this precious tool is also one of the most vulnerable parts of the human body, and the wrist joint is one of the most commonly injured in yoga.

Hand and Wrist Stretches

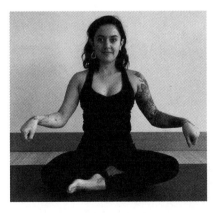

Simple Wrist Mobilization: Gently rotate the wrists through their full range of circular motion, repeatedly changing direction, then gently shake out the wrists for around thirty seconds. This can be incorporated in brief form into every Sun Salutation.

Wrist Pumps: Holding the fingers of one hand with the fingers of the other hand, move the wrist forward and back while resisting the movement with the opposing hand. Repeat for one to two minutes if pain-free.

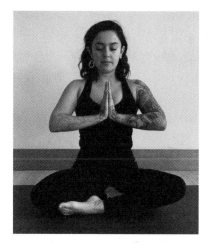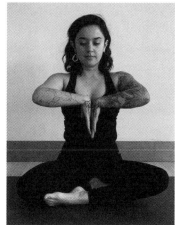

Anjali Mudra: Press the palms and fingers (from the knuckles to the fingertips) firmly together at the chest in a prayer position for one to two minutes. This is also known as the reverse Phalen's test; if there is a burning sensation inside the wrist joint within thirty seconds, this could indicate carpal tunnel syndrome. Reverse the position of the hands, placing the backs of the wrists and hands together, and press firmly for up to a minute (Phalen's test).

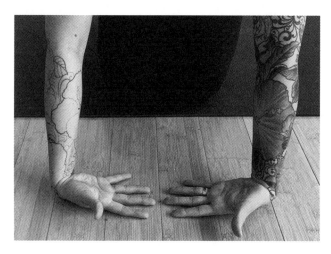

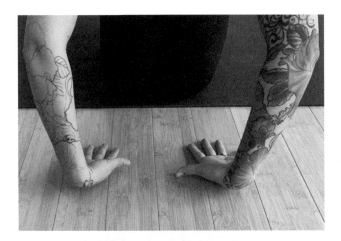

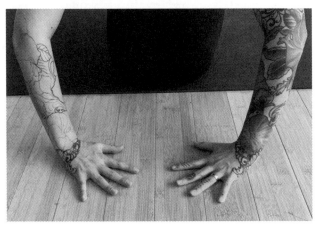

Hand Dance: Kneeling comfortably, place the hands down on the floor with the fingers pointed forward, then turn the palms up, then down with the fingers out, up with the fingers in, down with the fingers back, up with the fingers back, continuing in this fashion with every permutation of palms up and down with the fingers forward, back, in, and out.

Uttanasana Wrist Pratikriyasana: Whenever folding into Uttanasana amid Sun Salutations, place the backs of the wrists toward or onto the floor and make an easy fist. This is less intense on the wrists than Pada Hastasana (also, it can be easily done with the exhalation into Uttanasana).

The Neck

The colloquial euphemism "pain in the neck" refers to a persistent source of interpersonal annoyance. Looking more closely at the association of these two terms reveals a curious irony. "Pain," rooted in the Greek *poine,* "retribution, penalty," and Old French *peine,* "woe, suffering, punishment," is generally undesirable and may hurt. "Neck," rooted in the Old Germanic *hals,* "column," gave rise to the Middle English *halsen,* "to embrace or caress affectionately," which by the early nineteenth century in northern English dialect came to mean "to kiss, embrace," a generally desirable experience that may feel good. Pain and desire thus come together, albeit in a different way than is found in the heart of ancient yoga philosophies in which pain and suffering are posited as the inspiration for yoga and in which yoga is the path to freedom.

The neck is thus a place where one might experience much pleasure yet also a place perhaps most vulnerable to sudden trauma. In yoga asana practice, it is often in the hot pursuit of intensifying pleasure or joy in yoga or life that the neck is taken too quickly or too far in its safe ranges of motion or intrinsic pressure. In larger life, there is a vast array of sources of neck pain, including sleeping posture, prolonged posture, repetitive actions, spinal pathologies, emotional stress, arthritis, carotid artery dissection, thyroid cancer, esophageal trauma, and whiplash.

The primary focus of asanas in resolving muscular neck pain is to reduce muscular tension through proper skeletal alignment and the muscular stretching and strengthening that support it. A regular well-balanced general asana, pranayama, and meditation practice will help reduce the emotional stress often at the root of muscular neck tension. Most asanas involve sitting upright in the Simple Seated Pose or any comfortable sitting position, including in a chair, standing in Mountain Pose, or lying supine. The postures given here are described in a sitting position. To help sit comfortably tall, consider placing a block or bolster under your sitting bones.

Shoulder Rolls

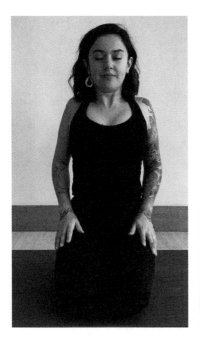 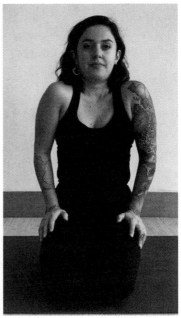

Special Sensitivity: Neck
Props: Block or bolster
Doing the Pose: Lift your shoulders up, back, down, forward and around several times, then go the opposite direction. Be very sensitive to pain; back off the movement if painful. Do this for one to two minutes.

Neck Stretch

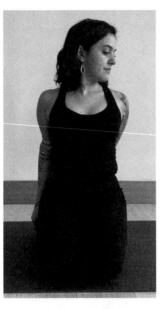

Special Sensitivity: Neck, shoulders
Props: None
Doing the Pose: Reach your left hand around your back to clasp your right arm above the elbow. Use your clasp to pull your right shoulder gently back and down. Turn your head toward your left shoulder. On your inhalations slightly lift your chin; on your exhalations draw your chin closer to your left shoulder. Hold for several breaths with your chin toward the shoulder and explore gingerly turning your head forward, drawing your ear toward your shoulder. Repeat several times before switching sides.

Step 3: Progressive Relaxation through Yoga Nidra

Overview

Although yoga nidra translates as "yoga sleep," the state of consciousness is akin to NREM stage N1 in which one is still aware of one's surroundings and sensations. Unlike simply (or not so simply!) slipping into unconscious sleep, in yoga nidra the thinking and reactive mind fades while awareness expands. It is, in its essence, a meditation practice and a practice of embodied awareness. It is also, by design, a very simple practice in which you scan your entire bodymind and progressively release tension.

The concept of yoga nidra as a state of consciousness is found in ancient texts (and discussed in part I). However, the practices of yoga nidra are a recent development in which yoga concepts and techniques are applied to progressive muscle relaxation, a stress-reduction modality developed and first published by Edmund Jacobson in 1929 while at Harvard University.[5] Yoga nidra also draws from the autogenic training developed by Johannes Heinrich Schultz in the early 1930s and the auto-suggestion techniques developed by Émile Coué in the early 1900s.[6] The beauty and power of what yoga nidra brings to progressive relaxation and autosuggestion techniques rest in yoga nidra being more focused on subtle awareness and accessing the deeper dimensions of consciousness than what relaxation and optimistic visualization accomplish alone, even as these are experienced and explored as entwined (especially when looked at through the prism of the koshas).

As with progressive relaxation, yoga nidra is guided in different ways by different teachers, some of whom insist that their method is the only true one because it somehow connects the dots of their view of yoga philosophy and the spiritual universe (so it is true to them!). There are also claims that when scanning the bodymind it must be done by tracing precise pathways mapped out by yogis thousands of years ago, despite such precise pathways never being so mapped by ancient yogis. The approach given here is more relaxed. It is about cultivating and thereby opening to the deepest possible relaxation and clear awareness. In doing so, the sequence begins in the face, then goes to the tips of your toes and up through your entire body.

The basic idea of Progressive Relaxation through Yoga Nidra is to be entirely wakeful in our awareness while utterly relaxed. The progressive relaxation might very well result in complete spontaneous pratyahara (i.e., you have fallen asleep), but the intention is to stay awake and attuned only to what you hear—mostly only the voice of your Progressive Relaxation through Yoga Nidra guide. The practice goes for about twenty to thirty minutes, or longer if you wish. It is ideal to do this practice with a guide. If possible, take yoga nidra classes, or use the free online audio practice at *www.markstephensyoga .com/resources/yoganidrameditation*. With practice you can do this independently. The following is a preview, with detailed instructions given immediately after.

You will begin lying down as though for Corpse Pose (Savasana) and relaxing everything as easily as you might, a sense of letting go of your senses except to hear. You will be invited to give yourself clear intention in the practice. For the next ten minutes or so, you will hear cues to feel and relax specific parts of your bodymind. The cues are given in quick succession so that there is no time to develop thoughts about them. The aim is to be mindful and feeling and releasing. This scanning will move from physical sensations (annamaya kosha) to breath awareness (pranamaya kosha) to thoughts and feelings (manomaya kosha) to more subtle sensations of intuitive awareness (vijnanamaya kosha) to feelings of complete ease and bliss (anandamaya kosha).

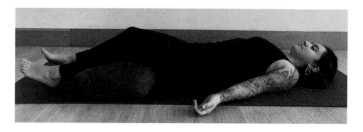

Special Sensitivity: The tendency to fall asleep
Props: Blankets, bolsters, eye pillow. Wear comfortable clothing. Choose a room that is quiet. Set the room temperature to be comfortable.

Doing the Yoga Nidra Sequence

Setting Up: Lie down on your back and position yourself as you would for Corpse Pose (Savasana). Place a rolled blanket or bolster under your knees for greater overall comfort and ease in your low back. Relax through your legs, allowing your feet to comfortably turn out. With your arms draped on the floor by your sides, rest the backs of your hands on the floor, letting your shoulders relax down. Cover your eyes with an eye pillow (ideally aroma-free). Once you are entirely comfortable, take several deep breaths in and allow the breath to freely release out, feeling your body settling into the floor.

Setting Intention: Your intention is important. Take a moment to reflect on your day, what is happening in your life, and what in this moment you most wish as the fruit of the practice. Giving yourself clearer intention, inner purpose, take a moment to breathe that intention into your heart, to better know it by heart.

Body Awareness (Annamaya Kosha): Allow your eyes to rest lightly closed, with a sense of softness around and through your eyes. Feel your temples and let the space between them lighten. Letting your tongue rest effortlessly in your mouth, relax your lips, let your jaw go lax and your throat soften. Bring your awareness to the tips of your right toes. Relax your right toes, from the little one across, one at a time, each toe letting go. Feel the sole of your foot relaxing, then the side and top of your foot, your heel, letting it soften. Sense your entire right foot relaxing. Now bring your awareness to the tips of your left toes. Relax your left toes, from the little one across, one at a time, each toe letting go. Feel the sole of your foot relaxing, then the side and top of your foot, your heel, letting it soften. Sense your entire left foot relaxing.

Feel your inner right ankle and relax it, now your outer right ankle and relax it. Feel your inner left ankle and relax it, now your outer left ankle and relax it. Feel your calves on the floor. Feel your right calf soften more into the floor, and let the bones and muscles through your lower right leg melt into your right calf. Feel your left calf soften more into the floor, and let the bones and muscles through your lower left leg melt into your left calf. Feel your entire lower legs as though heavier on the floor yet light within, as relaxed as can be in this moment.

Feel the back of your right knee and let it relax. Feel your inner right knee, letting it soften, your outer right knee softening, the front of your right knee softening. Feel the back of your left knee and let it relax. Feel your inner left knee, letting it soften, your outer left knee softening, the front of your left knee softening.

With your thighs resting on the floor, feel the back of your right thigh and let it relax. Feel your inner right thigh letting go, the top of your right thigh letting go, your outer right thigh completely relaxing. Feel the back of your left thigh and let it relax. Feel your inner left thigh letting go, the top of your left thigh letting go, your outer left thigh completely relaxing. Feel throughout both thighs, sensing them as releasing into the floor as relaxed as can be in this moment.

Feel your buttocks on the floor, the weight of your hips and pelvis releasing down. Bring your awareness to your right hip and let it soften. Relax your right buttock, the right side of your pelvis. Bring your awareness to your left hip and let it soften. Relax your left buttock, the left side of your pelvis. Feel your sacrum and the back of your pelvis resting effortlessly on the floor. Let go all through and around your pelvis.

Sense your belly effortlessly rising and falling with the effortless flow of the breath. Feel the right side of your abdomen and let it soften. Feel the left side of your abdomen and let it soften. Come to the center of your belly and let it completely relax. Feel your chest effortlessly rising and falling with the effortless flow of the breath. Feel the right side of your chest letting go, now the left side of your chest letting go, softening along your sternum and letting your collarbones spread apart. Allow the entire front of your torso to relax and sink as though into the back of your body.

Sensing your low back, relax to let it feel heavier on the floor. Feel the middle of your spine, your back ribs as though spreading and surrendering into the earth. Feel your right shoulder blade letting go, your left shoulder blade letting go, the space between your shoulder blades softening and relaxing. Sensing your chest, your heart center, open to the sky, let it let go, let your entire torso from front to back melt into the earth.

Bring your awareness to your right fingers. Focus on your right pinkie finger and let it relax. Feel your ring finger relax, your middle finger, index finger, and now your thumb all letting go. Relax through your right palm and let go between your right thumb and index finger. Bring your awareness to your left fingers. Focus on your left pinkie finger and let it relax. Feel your ring finger relax, your middle finger, index finger, and now your thumb all letting go. Relax through your left palm and let go between your left thumb and index finger. Let both of your hands and fingers rest lightly open toward the sky.

Feeling your right wrist, bring your awareness to the palm side of your right wrist and let it soften. Feel the back of your right wrist releasing toward the floor; let it. Feel your inner right forearm and relax it. Feel the outside of your right forearm on the floor, letting it go. Relax your right elbow to let it feel heavier on the floor. Feeling your left wrist, bring your awareness to the palm side of your left wrist and let it soften. Feel the back of your left wrist releasing toward the floor; let it. Feel your inner left forearm and relax it. Feel the outside of your left forearm on the floor, letting it go. Relax your left elbow to let it feel heavier on the floor. Feel your upper right arm and the front of it, your biceps, and let it go. Feel the back of your upper right arm and let it rest more fully onto the floor. Feel your upper left arm and the front of it, your biceps, and let it go. Feel the back of your upper left arm and let it rest more fully onto the floor. Now let both upper arms, forearms, wrists, hands, and fingers all surrender to the floor.

With your awareness in your neck, feel and relax the front of your neck. Feel the right side of your neck relaxing, the left side of your neck relaxing, the back of your neck relaxing. Bring your awareness back to your face. Let your jaw release, your mouth soften, your cheeks soften. Sensing your eyes resting lightly closed, allow a feeling of your eyes dropping back into your head, the space between your temples lighter and clearer. Feel your right ear and let it soften. Let your left ear soften. Feel the back of your head on the floor, and let it feel heavy. Sense the top of your head as soft as can be.

Feel your entire body fully supported on the floor. Allow the feeling of your body sinking down, tension draining away as though welcomed into the earth. With your awareness coming to the breath, sense with every effortless exhalation the deepening of your sense of calm and relaxation, a sense of the breath as though permeating all through your body, from your heart to the tips of your toes and fingers to the top of your head. For another moment just soak in that energy.

Breath Awareness (**Pranamaya Kosha**): Keeping your awareness in the breath, simply be with it, allowing it to flow in and out however it will. Sense the breath as it first touches your nostrils. Be just there with your awareness for a moment. Sense your belly and chest rising and falling with the flow of the breath. Just feel the movement with the flow of the breath. Allowing the breath to continue flowing effortlessly, start counting the breaths downward from 50 to 1. When the breath is flowing in, say to yourself, "belly rising 50," and as it flows out, say, "belly falling 50." Repeat this with 49, 48 ... eventually, 3, 2, 1.

If you lose count, continue from wherever you are. There is no such thing as making a mistake with this. The entire point is to be mindful of the breath, keeping your mind with the breath by aligning your words with the movement of your body that happens with the flow of the breath. Just keep coming back to watching, feeling, and counting the breaths. Amid this you will notice that your mind shifts to other thoughts. As soon as you notice other thoughts, come right back to the breath and your words to yourself. Keep going.

Return your awareness to the tips of your nostrils and again simply feel the breath flowing in and out. Still effortless in the movement of the breath, watch it, be with it when the sensation is at the openings of your nostrils. Once again count the breaths downward from 50 to 1. When the breath is flowing in, say to yourself, "nostrils opening 50," and as it flows out, say, "nostrils closing 50." Repeat this with 49, 48 ... eventually, 3, 2, 1.

To take this breathing practice further, start at 100 or 108. You can also start with a lower number and gradually begin higher. In practicing with the sensation of the breath at your nostrils, play with focusing in one round on the breath flowing in and out of your right nostril, then do a round focusing on the sensation in your left nostril. Use words as before: "inhaling right nostril 25, exhaling right nostril 25 ..."

Thoughts and Feelings Awareness (Manomaya Kosha): We are not our thoughts, even as it often seems we are led by our thoughts. Imagine your awareness before a thought arises, amid whatever thought is there, and after it has faded away: there you are, still aware, still you, regardless of thoughts or nonthoughts. Yet our thoughts can be powerful when we hold onto them, allowing them to magnify and become complicated. Imagine welcoming any thought in a way that it is just there, without attachment or interpretation, sensing it arising, noticing any emotions that come with it, recognizing any beliefs that come with it. Here the practice will be to gradually let a thought merely come and go along with the word that stimulates it, then another, then another, your emotions and mind present even as the words might evoke something inside of you. For example, the first word is "heartwarming." Upon hearing it, say it to yourself and be with whatever feeling is there. Then another word comes, and there you are, fully with it. This is a practice for training your mind to be with what is in the moment, not what came before, what might be, or that exists only in your imagination.

While breathing in let the thought arise and expand into your awareness, and while breathing out let it go. Visualize this happening as you now hear these words coming with the cycles of the breath, with a slight pause between each word. Hear it, say it to yourself, feeling whatever you are feeling, then another word will come.

Heartwarming, embarrassing, genius, challenge, easy, gripping, expensive, ridiculous, guilt, lazy, light, inspiring, serious, crave, delirious, begging, stunning, painless, painful, bold, hate, lunatic, practical, devastating, master, relentless, tempting, thrilling, frenzy, struggle, create, love, wild, weak, better, new, food, fool, dreamy, scared, silly, truth, intense, alive, hilarious, fantasy, hack, captivate, gorgeous, basic, weird, new, strange, suffer, ignite, shameful, joyful, ravenous, laughter, huge, quiet, relaxed.

Visualization (*Vijnanamaya Kosha*): Come back to sensing the breath, allowing it to flow freely and naturally. The words you will now hear will stimulate your imagination. Let them. Notice where they take you, where you take you. If you are not familiar with what the words denote, let your imagination run free. Be present to just the words and the impressions they cause in your awareness.

Imagine 1: The Sahara Desert, the Eiffel Tower, the moon, a cloudy sky, a newborn baby, a blue car, the Golden Gate Bridge, a river, a towering redwood tree, the ocean, the sky, a sunrise, a skyscraper, a luscious jungle, a rainbow, your heart.

Imagine 2: Keep your awareness in your heart for a moment. Imagine the breath flowing in and out through the middle of your chest, your spiritual heart center. As the breath is flowing effortlessly in, imagine it as warm light flowing into the innately spacious love in your heart. As the breath flows out, imagine it fading out behind you as though the wake of a boat. Breathing in through your heart, imagine breathing pain into your heart, feeling it in your heart. As the breath flows out, sense that pain fading out as if into the wake of the breath behind you. Stay present with the breath, and imagine or sense what pain you have. Breathing in through your heart, imagine breathing that pain even more deeply into your heart. As the breath flows out, sense that pain fading out as if into the wake of the breath behind you. Do this again, breathing in a deeper layer of that pain into the infinitely spacious love in your heart, and just as easily let it go. Breathing in through your heart, imagine breathing what you most fear into the infinitely spacious love in your heart, and just as easily let it go. Do it again, present to the feeling of fear coming into your heart, present to that feeling fading away. Breathing in through your heart, imagine breathing in what makes you most joyful, and just as easily let it go. Do it again. Be with joy, and let it go, and just be back in the breath, resting in the freedom of your imagination.

Imagine 3: Imagine the space at the base of your spine, your root chakra, *muladhara,* and imagine the foundation of your being as balanced as can be, having what you need, unconcerned with your needs, at peace with your place in the world. Imagine light slowly rising from that space into your lower navel, the *svadisthana chakra,* the source place of your creativity. Focusing on that place, imagine feeling safe and free in all the ways you creatively express yourself in life, from how you prepare food to how you love and care for yourself and others. Imagine the balance of your creative energies in ways that allow them to be freer, more open, more aligned with all you value. Imagine the light from that place rising into your belly, your awareness coming to the *manipura chakra,* the city of gems, the space where willfulness originates and manifests. Imagine your inner fire perfectly tended, neither so hot that it burns you out or causes aggression nor so dim that you are timid. Imagine from the balance of energy in your muladhara, svadisthana, and manipura chakras flowing into your heart, to your *anahata chakra.* Sensing the breath flowing through your heart, imagine love, imagine loving and being loved in the most amazing ways, that love, this love radiating into every aspect of your life. Imagine the light, warmth, and love in your heart flowing into your throat, your *vishudda chakra,* your voice sweet and kind, your words easy to say and easy for others to hear. Imagine the light flowing into your head, your *ajna chakra,* and imagine seeing out as though through the center of your forehead, seeing and sensing everything as clearly as can be. Imagine being filled with this warm and clear light, from the tips of your toes through the crown of your head, your *sahasrara chakra.* Imagine the crown of your head opening to the universe, the light within you connecting with the light of the universe. Present, whole, at peace, here you are.

*Affirmation (**Anandamaya Kosha**)*: Feel your body, your contact with the floor. Sense the breath, your body as though being breathed by the breath. Allow your whole body to be breathed and to relax. Imagine being utterly at peace, a sense of deep and abiding equanimity all through and around you. Imagine joy, be in that joy, enjoy. Let it soak in for several cycles of breath.

Changing as little as possible, come back to the intention you gave yourself at the beginning of this practice. Revisiting it, perhaps renewing it, begin to breathe a little more deeply and consciously. Come back to feeling sensation throughout your body, breathing as though down into your toes, to reawaken everywhere, everything. Take a moment to give yourself clear intention for what comes next, rising from the floor, sitting, doing whatever you will do.

This is a great time to simply sit quietly for a few minutes. If it is time for bed, go to bed. If not, do a quiet, calm activity, keep the light dim, and be in your bliss.

Chapter
6

YOGA SLEEP SEQUENCE FOR DEPRESSION OR LETHARGY

Introduction: Depression, Sleep, and Brightening Your Day

Sleep and depression are intertwined: poor sleep exacerbates depression and depression exacerbates poor sleep; improved sleep contributes to improved mood and improved mood contributes to improved sleep. This points to a path on which sleep and mood are both directly addressed.

As human beings, we experience a wide range of emotional states, including qualities of sadness, melancholia, and anhedonia that are typically labeled as depression, and as such considered unhealthy, even when they are moderate and are normal responses to life events. The same life events can also lead to a state of deep uneasiness and apprehension characteristic of anxiety, giving us the entwined condition of dysthymic disorder. The clinical diagnosis of depression considers the severity and persistence of specific symptoms such as sadness, overarching hopelessness or pessimism, irritability, loss of interest in what were once pleasurable activities, suicidal ideation, or difficulty sleeping, eating, or working. The technical definition of "depression" given in the *DSM-V* distinguishes persistent depressive disorder (a depressed mood that lasts at least two years), from perinatal depression (also known as postpartum melancholia), psychotic depression (involving some form of psychosis), and seasonal affective disorder (winter depression brought on by diminished sunlight). There is a vast array of conditions and experiences within each of these types of depression that can be episodic or so habitual that they come to form a core part of someone's sense of self. As we saw in chapter 2, these conditions are often associated with insomnia and other sleep disorders.

Depression can be caused by a wide array of factors, starting with the conditions of one's life during childhood, particularly abandonment, physical abuse, and sexual abuse.[1] Many life events—some of which are less "events" than lifelong experiences—can trigger a depressive reaction: illness, major life changes, the experience of living in a racist, sexist, ageist, or otherwise discriminatory society, financial difficulty, violence, loss, social isolation, and difficult social relationships. Drug abuse—even simple use of some substances and certainly the use of a wide array of FDA-approved medications—can cause or exacerbate mood disorders. There are also physiological factors that can create chemical imbalances in the brain that cause emotional depression.

Most depression passes with time, especially when one is capable of being active, shares time with and confides in others, and avoids known triggers. When depression is persistent or is experienced with other conditions such as acute anxiety or substance abuse, this may indicate the value of treatment. The most common treatments for depression are some form of psychotherapy, particularly cognitive behavioral therapy, and antidepressant medication, often in combination.[2] Seemingly every form of alternative and complementary therapy offers something for healing depression.[3] Mindfulness-based meditation as a tool in cognitive therapy has gained significant traction as an effective method for reducing depression across a wide spectrum of settings.[4] There is also increasing evidence for the efficacy of other meditation practices, including Vipassana, in healing depression.[5] Although there are many claims made about the effectiveness of yoga in healing depression, there are few high-quality studies supporting this assertion.[6]

The *Yoga Sūtra* sets out the basic purpose of yoga as chitta vrtti nirodha, "to calm the fluctuations of the mind." From the late twentieth century to the present we find numerous elaborations and refinements of this idea as it pertains to mental health,[7] and very recently evidence of success in using specific yoga practices for healing depression and anxiety.[8] The heart of yoga for healing depression rests in opening to self-acceptance while walking a path of life-changing practices. The embodiment practices of asana can help bring us into the present moment, thereby reducing the tendency to dwell on earlier life events or to obsess about something that has not yet happened.

Depression is most commonly just that—a depressed condition in which one feels low energy, lack of interest in what were once enjoyable activities, and sometimes physical pain arising from compression in some parts of the body. Thus, such low-energy depression can be described in yogic terms as *tamasic* depression. But although we might think of depression as feeling "down," depression can also manifest with anxiety, anger, and restlessness, even as one feels hopeless, in yogic terms a *rajasic* depression. Such a mixed affective state calls for a delicate balance of calming and stimulating practices, while if more tamasic or more rajasic, the practices should be relatively more stimulating or more calming. Where one has rajasic depression, or a combination of depression and anxiety, this points to alternating between the Yoga Sleep Sequence for Hyperarousal in chapter 5 and the Yoga Sleep Sequence for Depression or Lethargy described below.

As discussed in chapter 3 regarding somatics and consciousness, yoga asana practice can be a tool for reexperiencing the bodymind in affirmative ways, rooting out embodied negative emotions while rendering a more peaceful and joyful bodymind. The basic idea is that each moment in any asana is experienced as though we are opening so many different windows onto our tendencies in life, which allows us to see ourselves more clearly through the various thoughts and feelings that arise in reaction to an asana in that immediate moment.

Unless anxious, when depressed we tend to take on a depressed posture. Rather than using grounding actions through our feet and legs to stand tall, we tend to sink into our skeleton. Rather than rooting our sitting bones when sitting, we tend to slump. Rather than being open across our chest, we tend to collapse our chest, unconsciously creating the universal human sign of emotional depression. We also tend to dwell in our thoughts about what has happened in the past and what might happen in the future, this in contrast to being present in the current moment. We can counter these tendencies with postural practices that reveal and affirm the value of active grounding, a tall spine, and an open heart. There is also value in approaching the postural practice with dynamic movement that is mildly stimulating and that naturally invites being more present in the moment and thus less inclined to go into habitually negative thoughts and emotions.

When we add breathing practices, starting with basic ujjayi pranayama and asana, we can play with the ways in which qualities of breathing affect qualities of self-awareness. While taking in breath, we tend to sense more expansive awareness, a greater and lighter space inside in which there is great potential for deeper personal insight. As we release the breath, we tend to settle, calm, and quiet down inside, especially in the natural pause that occurs when empty of breath. Staying in a simple breath-focused meditation practice (described in chapter 4) can allow us to gradually let go of self-limiting and self-destructive patterns of mental and emotional reactions to life events, even as we might still find ourselves exposed to the very triggers that otherwise cause depressive episodes. Thus, it is in the blended practices of asana, pranayama, and meditation that we attain the most healing effects of yoga for depression and insomnia.

In doing this sequence, try to follow the order of postures as given here. Omit any that you cannot do with stability and ease.

Experienced yoga students can substitute a steadily flowing and stimulating yoga practice (emphasizing standing and back-bending postures) such as Vinyasa flow for the Dynamic Postural Practice given here. More than fifty flowing-style practices designed for varying levels of ability and different physical foci are provided in *Yoga Sequencing: Designing Transformative Yoga Classes.*

When to Do the Yoga Sleep Sequence for Depression or Lethargy

- In the morning or early afternoon
- If you do it in the evening, omit step 2 and do the postures given in chapter 4's "Basic Yoga Sleep Sequence" after the sequence given here.

What You Will Need

- Two or three blankets folded into a rectangular form about three feet wide by two feet deep
- One or two large bolsters, cushions, or pillows
- One or two yoga blocks (or very thick books)
- A yoga mat or large rug

Doing the Sequence

Step 1: Dynamic Postural Practice

Tuning In: Come to standing at the front of your yoga mat. If you would like, draw your palms together at your heart and take several deep breaths as though in and out through the middle of your chest. Bring your fingertips to your forehead; reflecting, give yourself clearer intention in this practice, then bring your hands back to your heart and breathe your intention into your heart, giving yourself a sense of knowing it by heart.

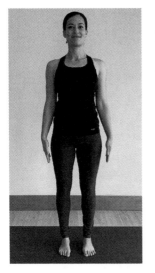

Ujjayi Pranayama: Changing as little as possible in your comfort and the flow of the breath, open your mouth and breathe out as though you are trying to breathe fog onto a glass or mirror. In doing so, sense the breath in your throat and how when it flows over your vocal cords it gives the breath a light whisper-like sound. Maintain this sound and sensation of the breath in your throat as you draw the breath in. Do this for three cycles of breath. Now keep breathing with this sound and sensation but with your mouth closed, using the sensations of the breath to make it smoother and simpler. Breathe with this ujjayi—uplifting—technique throughout this practice.

Mountain to Upward Arms to Mountain

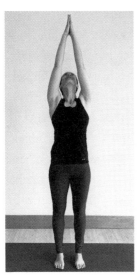

Special Sensitivity: Low back, shoulders, neck

Props: None

Doing the Pose: Rather than a static "pose," this is a dynamic movement done in coordination with the breath. Standing tall with your feet hip-distance apart, actively root down through your feet, bringing more length to your spine, and extend through your arms and fingers as though reaching them to the floor. Completely exhaling, turn your hands outward. On the inhalation, slowly reach your arms outward and upward until your palms touch overhead. It is okay if your palms do not come together. On the exhalation, turn your palms outward and slowly reach your arms outward and downward until they are at your sides (or continue this movement by bringing your palms back together at your heart). In repeating this movement ten times, keep your legs strongly engaged (firming your thigh muscles), rooting your feet, and standing tall up through your spine. When moving your arms, reach out through your arms and fingers as strongly as you comfortably can; in doing so, visualize energy radiating from your heart through your fingertips and beyond. If it is comfortable for your neck, raise your gaze up as you raise your arms; otherwise, look forward.

Breath of Joy

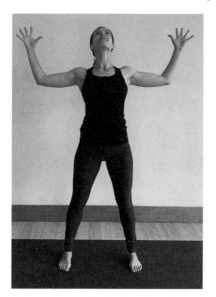

Special Sensitivity: Shoulders, neck

Props: None

Doing the Pose: Standing with your feet hip-distance apart or wider, bring your fingertips to your chest with your elbows lifted level with your shoulders. On each inhalation, reach your arms out and back, expanding across your chest while raising your gaze. On each exhalation, draw your fingertips back to your chest, rounding your upper back while bringing your gaze toward your heart. Explore doing this with much deeper breathing. Repeat ten to fifteen times.

Inner Fire

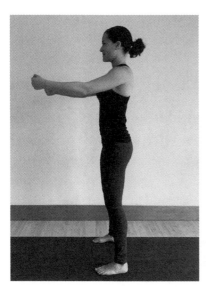 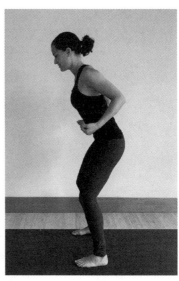

Special Sensitivity: Neck, shoulders

Props: None

Doing the Pose: Standing with your feet hip-distance apart or wider, on the inhalation reach both arms forward with your palms turned upward. On each exhalation, strongly and quickly pull your arms back while bending your elbows and making tight fists. As you inhale and extend your arms, gaze slightly up; as you exhale and pull your arms back, gaze toward your belly. While using ujjayi pranayama in creating the inhalations, on the exhalations open your mouth and make a strong and lengthened "haaa" sound. Repeat ten to fifteen times, then shake out your arms and take a moment to relax and let the effects soak in.

Tree Pose

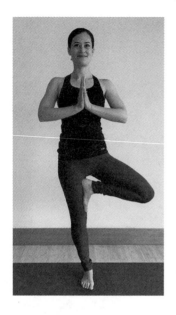

Special Sensitivity: Knees (especially in the standing leg)

Props: If necessary, use a wall for support.

Doing the Pose: Start in Mountain Pose. If necessary, use the wall for support. If possible, place the heel of the lifted leg high up in the inner thigh of the standing leg. If unable to place the foot above the knee, place it below the knee (on the inner calf or ankle). At first, keep the hands on the hips or at the heart; try to maintain even hips, pelvic neutrality, and abduction of the lifted leg as you try to press the bent knee back. If steady, raise the arms and explore looking up. Release slowly.

Triangle Pose

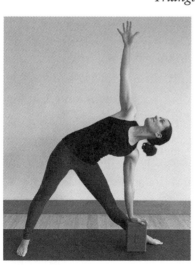

Special Sensitivity: Knee of front leg, neck, low back

Props: Block, wall (if necessary for balance)

Doing the Pose: Start with the feet separated the length of one leg; turn the left foot out ninety degrees, and turn the right foot slightly in. Shift the hips to the right, pressing the left sitting bone toward the right heel while reaching out to the left through the spine and arm to the point of maximum extension, then release the hand onto the lower leg or ankle. Consider looking down to make it easier on the neck. Consider initially bringing the hand higher up the shin to ease the lengthening and slight rotation of the spine. The legs are straight and strong without hyperextending the knees; the front leg's kneecap is lifted and pointed forward. Try to lengthen through the spine. Being sensitive to the neck, consider *not* looking up.

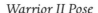

Warrior II Pose

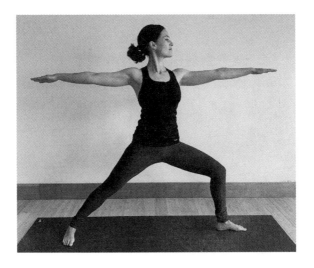

Special Sensitivity: Knee of front leg, shoulders, neck
Props: None
Doing the Pose: Start in a Wide-Angle Forward Fold stance, turning the left foot out, turning the right foot slightly in, slowly bending the left knee while guiding it toward the outside of the foot; if the knee goes beyond the heel, crawl the toes farther forward for a longer stance. If starting from the Warrior I Pose, keep the left-knee alignment while pressing the right thigh back.

The left knee is aligned directly above the heel (it will tend to splay in); the left sitting bone draws under; hips are level, pelvis neutral, right leg firm with the arch lifted; shoulder blades are down the back; energy runs up through the spine and out from the heart center through the fingertips. Press through the feet to release.

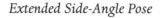

Extended Side-Angle Pose

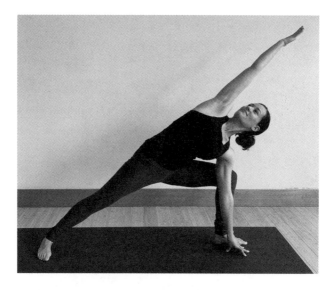

Special Sensitivity: Knees, back ankle, low back, neck, upper shoulder

Props: Block

Doing the Pose: From the Warrior II Pose, keep the feet grounded and reach out through the right arm and side, initially placing the left elbow on the left knee. Drawing the shoulder blades down the back, revolve the torso open, reach the right arm down the right leg, turn the palm up to feel the external rotation of the arm, then reach the arm overhead. Over time, bring the left fingertips or palm to a block or the floor to the inside of the left foot, and over time to the outside of the foot. Minimize lateral flexion of the spine while rotating the torso open. Maintain a strong line of energy from the grounded right foot through the extended fingertips. Press the left elbow or shoulder against the knee to keep the knee aligned and to leverage rotation of the torso. Gaze to the right fingertips or relax the neck and look across the room or to the floor.

Half Moon

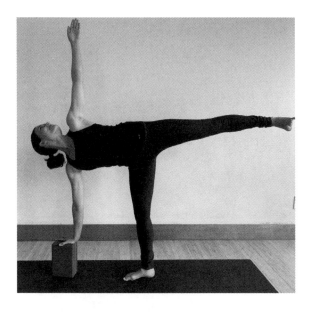

Special Sensitivity: Standing ankle and knee, low back, neck
Props: Block, wall
Doing the Pose: Transition in stages from Triangle Pose (described above) by bending the front knee, placing the fingertips about a foot in from the front foot (on the floor or on a block), sliding the back foot closer to the front foot until fully weighting the front foot and hand, then slowly beginning to straighten the front leg while keeping the back hip rotated fully open. Another

method of transitioning into Half Moon is to tip to the side from standing, holding a block in the lower hand; first try this with your back to a wall. Maintain external rotation of the hips while transitioning; keep the standing foot from turning in; extend the lifted leg straight back from the hip; radiate out from the belly through the legs and spine; and from the heart center radiate out through the fingertips.

Cat-Dog

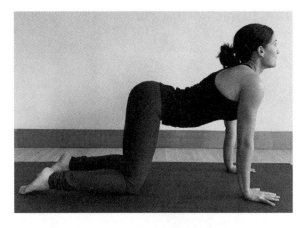

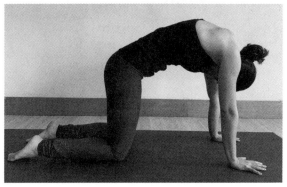

Special Sensitivity: Wrists, neck, spine
Props: None

Doing the Pose: Come onto all fours, aligning your wrists under your shoulders (or slightly ahead of your shoulders if you have tender wrists) and your knees under your hips, hip-distance apart. With each inhalation, slowly rotate your pelvis forward to raise your sitting bones while creating a feeling of pulling your chest forward as though through your arms (if it is okay with your neck, look slightly up). With each exhalation, reverse this positioning by arching your back to the sky like a cat, pulling your forehead and pelvis toward each other. Repeat five to ten times.

Puppy Dog

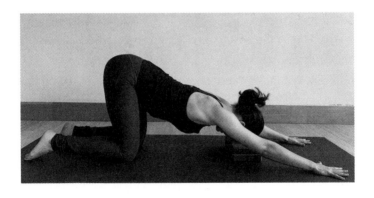

Special Sensitivity: Neck, low back, shoulders
Props: None
Doing the Pose: Begin on all fours with your wrists under your shoulders and your knees under your hips. Reach your arms forward from your shoulders and press your hands firmly and evenly into the floor. Try to rotate your shoulder blades out away from your spine. With each inhalation, lift your chest up away from the floor. With each exhalation, stretch your chest toward the floor. Repeat ten to fifteen times before holding your chest toward the floor for up to two minutes.

Downward Facing Dog

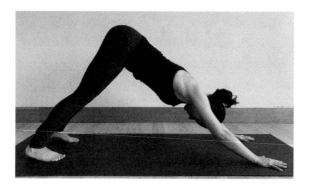

Special Sensitivity: Wrists, shoulders, hamstrings, neck

Props: None

Doing the Pose: This pose stretches and strengthens several parts of the body, mostly through the arms, shoulders, legs, and hips. Ultimately, it helps to lengthen the spine. From all fours, curl your toes under and try to rotate your pelvis forward (lifting your sitting bones). With firm pressure through your hands (try to press down the knuckles of your forefingers), slowly lift your hips up while gradually straightening your legs. If you have difficulty straightening your legs, play with a wider foot stance; it is okay to keep your knees bent, too. When you first come into the pose, play with bicycling your legs and twisting through your torso, thereby more easily feeling your way into the pose by releasing initial tension. Pressing through your hands, try to roll your shoulder blades out away from your spine. If it is okay with your neck, align your ears with your arms so your neck is in its natural form. Firm your thighs and press the tops of your thighs back to lengthen your spine. Start with holding this pose for a few breaths, rest on all fours for a few breaths, then come into it, gradually extending the time you hold this pose for up to two minutes. Rest on all fours or in Child's Pose.

Handstand

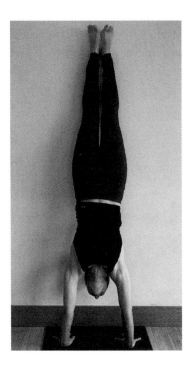

Special Sensitivity: Hands, wrists, elbows, shoulders, low back
Props: Wall
Doing the Pose: Begin in Downward Facing Dog. Extend one leg back and up, keeping it straight and strong; begin springing off the other foot while swinging the lifted leg up. The moment the springing leg is sprung, make it straight and strong, and draw it up next to the other leg overhead. Pressing down firmly through the hands as in Downward Facing Dog, first flex the feet and extend up through the legs and heels, then point and press out through the balls of the feet. While lengthening through the core of the body, wrap the shoulder blades broadly as in Downward Facing Dog, lightly engage the belly to support the stable connection of the torso and pelvis, keep the floating ribs in and

away from the skin while pressing the tailbone and pelvis up, lift from the floor of your pelvis, spiral the femurs internally, and breathe while gazing down between the thumbs. Hold for up to one minute. Slowly release one leg down at a time, then either rest in Child's Pose or in a standing forward fold for several seconds before rising up to standing.

Locust

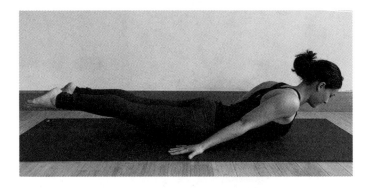

Special Sensitivity: Low back, neck
Props: None
Doing the Pose: Lie prone with your palms facing the floor. Pressing your hips and feet firmly into the floor, create a feeling of radiating energy down through your legs and feet while slightly pressing your tailbone toward your heels. Maintain this active engagement of your legs. On each inhalation, slowly and slightly lift your chest off the floor, keeping your ears aligned with your shoulders so your neck is in its natural form. If it is comfortable for your low back, lift your legs at the same time. On each exhalation, slowly and steadily release everything to the floor. In repeating this movement four to five times, explore lifting slightly higher each time. The fifth time you lift off the floor, stay lifted, interlace your fingers behind your back, and

lift your arms up away from your back, thereby increasing the stretch across your chest. Hold for five to ten breaths before very slowly releasing back to the floor. Explore repeating Locust two to three times.

Bow

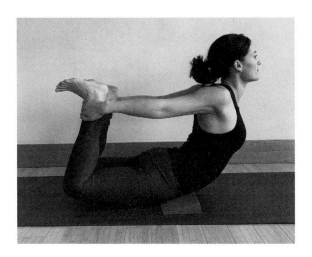

Special Sensitivity: Low back, shoulders
Props: Blanket or wedge
Doing the Pose: Lying prone, bend your knees and reach back to clasp your ankles. Flex your ankles to stabilize your knees. Rooting down through your hips, pull on your ankles to lift your chest and the legs up off the floor, pressing your tailbone back while spreading across your collarbones. Try to rock back farther onto your thighs to lift your chest higher, then press your feet back up. Focus the backbend in your mid-spine. Hold for five to ten breaths. If it is difficult to bring your knees toward the floor (to rock back onto your thighs), slightly elevate the top of your hips onto a folded blanket or a wedge. If unable to clasp your ankles, do Bridge instead.

Bridge

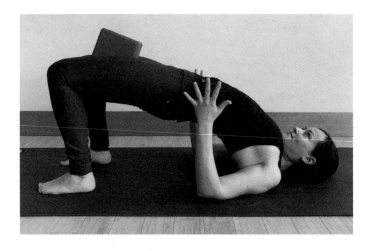

Special Sensitivity: Low back, neck, knees, shoulders
Props: Blankets, block
Doing the Pose: Lying supine, slide your feet in close to your but-tocks, hip-distance apart and parallel. With completion of each exhalation, feel your lower back press toward the floor and your tailbone curl up; this is the action that you will use to initiate the lift into Bridge. With the inhalation, press through your feet to lift your hips up while pressing your tailbone toward your knees (maintaining space in your low back). Bend your elbows, pointing your fingers up, then press your elbows firmly down into the floor to expand more across your chest. Either main-tain this arm position, or interlace your fingers under your back and shrug your shoulders slightly under, just enough to draw any pressure off your neck. Press down firmly through the feet to keep lifting your hips. Pressing down through your shoul-ders, elbows, and wrists, press the tips of your shoulder blades in toward your heart while lifting the sternum toward your chin and spreading broadly across your upper back and collarbones.

Hold for one to two minutes. To release, lift your heels, reach your arms overhead, and slowly roll down one vertebra at a time. Repeat one to two times. If there is pressure on the back of your neck when in Bridge, place blankets under your back and shoulders.

Wheel

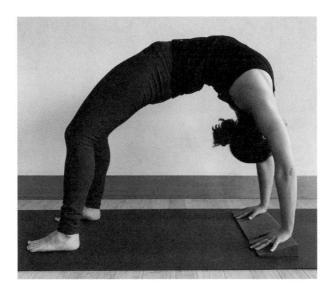

Special Sensitivity: Low back, wrists, shoulders, knees
Props: Wedge
Doing the Pose: Start as for Bridge with your feet parallel and close to your hips. Place your palms on the floor by and in line with your shoulders. Position your elbows to point straight up; if unable to do this, play with separating your hands a little wider and turning your fingertips slightly out to ease the external rotation, creating a feeling of sliding your palms back to root your shoulder blades against your back ribs. If the positioning of your hands and elbows is difficult, play with placing your hands on a

wedge. With an inhalation, press onto the top of your head with your hips lifted off the floor to reaffirm the positioning of your elbows and shoulders. With another inhalation, press your arms as straight as you can. Maintain active legs, and lengthen your tail-bone toward your knees. Press evenly down through your hands. Hold for five to ten breaths. Repeat one to two times.

Knees to Chest

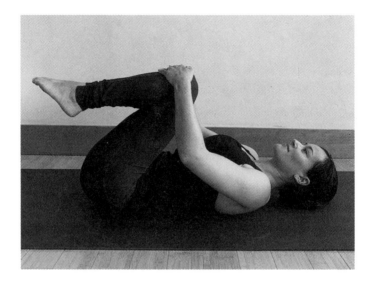

Special Sensitivity: Knees, low back
Props: None
Doing the Pose: Lying on your back, slide your feet in toward your hips, then clasp your knees to draw them in toward your chest. With each inhalation, release your knees away from your chest. With each exhalation, draw them in a little closer. If you feel pressure in your knees, clasp behind them so they do not fully bend. Play with this movement for one to two minutes, releasing tension around your upper legs and hips, and in your low back.

Supine Twist

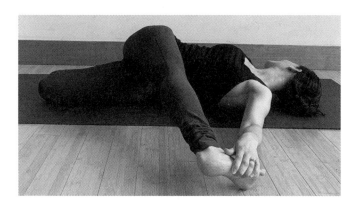

Special Sensitivity: Low back, knees
Props: Blocks
Doing the Pose: Lying supine with your knees in toward your chest, stretch your left leg straight out onto the floor. Draw your right knee across your body to come into a twist through your torso. If you have low back issues or feel tension in your low back, keep your knees bent and place a block between your knees and/or under the lower knee before twisting. Be more interested in keeping your shoulders on the floor than getting the knee to the floor. Switch sides.

Resting Cobbler

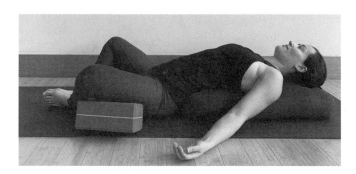

Special Sensitivity: Knees, inner thighs, low back
Props: Block, bolsters, folded blankets, sandbags
Doing the Pose: Set up for Cobbler as described in chapter 5, with folded blankets or bolsters stacked behind you. Slowly recline back with your hands on the floor behind you, easing your back and head onto the blankets or bolsters. Place blocks under your knees if there is intense pressure in the inner knees or thighs. If you want a deeper stretch, place sandbags on your knees.

Spacious Heart

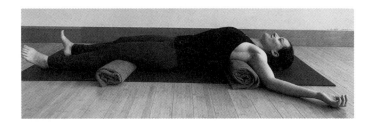

Special Sensitivity: Low back, neck
Props: Bolsters, blankets
Doing the Pose: Preparing to lie supine, place a rolled blanket and one or two bolsters on your mat. Lying over the props, place the rolled blanket under your knees and the bolsters under your back (sensitive to your low back) with your buttocks on the floor. Release your arms to the floor by your sides. Relax in this form for five minutes.

Step 2: Energizing and Emotionally Balancing Breathing Practice

Kapalabhati Pranayama: Cultivating Light

Note: This practice is contraindicated if you are anxious, have high blood pressure or a heart condition, or are pregnant.

Kapalabhati (from *kapala*, "skull," and *bhati*, "luster") *pranayama* energizes the entire body and creates a feeling of exhilaration. In natural breathing, the inhalation is active—that is, it is activated by muscles—whereas the exhalation is passive, resulting from contraction of the elastic lungs. This is reversed in kapalabhati pranayama: the exhalations are made active and inhalations passive.

1. Start by doing several rounds of ujjayi pranayama, warming and awakening the lungs while activating *mula bandha* (lightly lifting the pelvic floor).

2. After completion of an ujjayi exhalation, draw in the breath halfway and then rapidly and repeatedly blast it out through the nose, with a slight pause when empty of breath. The sound is in the nostrils, not the throat.

3. The inhalation happens naturally.

4. In the early development of this practice, do twenty-five rapid exhalations, then fill your lungs and hold the breath in for a few counts before releasing the breath and relaxing.

5. After this and each successive round, draw your attention to the sensations you feel in your head, perhaps sensing the calming and clearing effects of this practice.

6. Gradually increase to several minutes of sustained kapalabhati.

7. Complete the kapalabhati practice with Savasana.

Bhastrika Pranayama: The Fiery Bellows Breath

Note: This practice is contraindicated if you are anxious, have high blood pressure or a heart condition, or are pregnant.

Bhastrika ("bellows") *pranayama* is similar to kapalabhati, though more intense in fanning the flames of inner fire. Explore this technique only after you are comfortable in the kapalabhati practice. Here both the inhalations and exhalations are done through the nostrils vigorously and in rapid succession. Unlike kapalabhati, there is no pause after the exhalation.

1. Start sitting and doing ujjayi pranayama.

2. Initiate bhastrika by quickly blasting out the breath after a half inhalation.

3. Make the following inhalation just as strong and quick as the exhalation, followed by a strong and quick exhalation, completing one round of bhastrika. The sound should come from the nose, not the throat.

4. Do five to ten rounds, ending with an exhalation and several rounds of ujjayi pranayama, then repeat three or more times.

5. Gradually increase the number of cycles in each round and the number of rounds in each sitting, eventually sustaining bhastrika for five to ten minutes.

6. Rest in Savasana.

Sitali Pranayama: Cooling Breath

The purpose of *sitali* ("cooling") *pranayama* is to cool and calm the physical body and mind. It can be done at any time, including during asana practice and after fiery pranayamas such as kapalabhati. Here the tongue is extended slightly out of the mouth, and its sides are curled up to form a channel. (The ability to create this channel is genetic; some people can do it, others cannot. If you cannot curl your tongue, visualize the curling and continue with the practice.) Explore as follows:

1. Sitting comfortably, close the eyes and relax.

2. Extend the tongue and curl its sides to create a channel for moisture.

3. Slowly and deeply draw in the breath across the tongue, sensing the breath becoming moist and cool as it passes across the tongue.

4. Then close the mouth and slowly exhale through the nose.

5. Repeat this ten times, then relax.

6. Gradually build up the sitali pranayama practice for up to fifteen minutes.

Suryabheda Pranayama: Stimulating Vitality

Suryabheda (from surya, "sun," and bheda, "to pierce") pranayama is said to pierce the pingala nadi and activate pranic energy. The pingala nadi is said to receive prana through the right nostril. In suryabheda pranayama, the fingers are applied to the nostrils to regulate the breath:

1. Sit comfortably and do several rounds of ujjayi pranayama.

2. Draw the fingers to the nostrils as described in the following "Nadi Shodhana Pranayama" section, blocking the left nostril.

3. Inhale slowly and deeply through the right nostril, close both nostrils, and hold the breath in for a few seconds.

4. Open the left nostril, and exhale slowly and completely.

5. This completes one cycle of suryabheda pranayama. Repeat for up to thirty minutes, followed by Savasana.

Nadi Shodhana Pranayama: Alternate Nostril Breathing

This practice is said to harmonize the hemispheres of the brain.

1. Sit comfortably and practice ujjayi pranayama for a few minutes.

2. Place the fingertips on one side of the nose, the thumb on the other side, just below the slight notch about half-way down the side of the nose. Try to place the fingers with even pressure on the left and right sides of the nose, maintaining steady contact while keeping the nostrils fully open.

3. While continuing ujjayi pranayama, play with slightly varying the pressure of the fingers, becoming more sensitive to the effects of the fine finger adjustments.

4. After a complete exhalation, close the right nostril and slowly inhale through the left.

5. At the crest of the inhalation, close the left nostril and slowly exhale through the right.

6. Empty of breath, fully inhale through the right, close the right, and exhale through the left.

7. Continue with this initial form of alternate nostril breathing for up to five minutes, cultivating the smooth and steady flow of the breath while remaining relaxed and calm.

Step 3: Heart-Centered Meditation

Sitting comfortably, draw your palms together at your heart in anjali mudra, the reverence seal. Bring your awareness to the breath and allow it to be as light and simple as can be. Simply be with the breath for about a minute.

Feeling your contact with the floor, imagine energy rising from the base of your spine and out through the crown of your head. Imagine this energy like warm white light beaming out toward the sky. With your awareness resting in the effortless flow of breath, keeping your palms together, with an inhalation raise your palms up past your face and slowly overhead as though through that beam of light, grounding down while reaching toward the sky, spaciousness all through you. As you exhale, slowly extend your arms out and down, a sense of drawing that light out and around you as you bring the backs of your hands to rest softly on your knees, with a sense of being warmly enveloped as though in a cocoon of nourishing light.

Staying with the breath, spread your fingers and palms wide open, a sense of radiating energetically from your heart center out through your fingertips and the crown of your head. Bringing the tips of your thumbs and index fingers together into *jnana mudra (the basic meditative hand position)*, let your thumbs symbolize all that you consider divine or beautiful in the universe, your index fingers all that is divine or beautiful in yourself, the touching of your thumbs and fingertips representing that yoking, the union, the whole of these qualities—of *you*.

Breathing and following the natural flow of the breath, allow the three extended fingers on each hand to represent your release of the difficulties in your life that keep you from feeling more whole, happy, and complete—letting fear, anger, and any unhealthy attachments give way to contentment, self-acceptance, and love. Staying in the light of this awareness, keep following the breath, breath by effortless breath creating a sense of deepening self-awareness and self-acceptance in this perfect moment.

Chapter

7

BETTER SLEEP FOR YOUNG AND OLD

Sleeping through the Ages

The biology and timing of sleep change across our lifetime. There are unique sleep issues present at every age, with natural sleep timing and sleep time requirements varying by age and to some extent by individual.[1] Here we focus on better sleep for children (infants, toddlers, and school-age children), adolescents, and older adults. Regarding children, especially infants and toddlers, the guidance here is for parents, while we offer separate yoga practices for older children, adolescents, and older adults. Depending on one's conditions, the practices given in earlier and later chapters can be done in conjunction with the guidance given for those with sleep problems in these phases of life.

Children's Sleep

Fetuses are rarely awake, as their sleeping brain, mostly in REM sleep, is working intensively to wire itself. (Most of the movement a mother feels her unborn baby making results from the baby's lack of muscle atonia.) Infants continue to mostly sleep—polyphasically, as they frequently awaken—because their brain is rapidly developing, with frequent sleep disturbance in infants (including from a nursing mother's alcohol, caffeine, or nicotine consumption) associated with autism.[2] Their sleep finally starts to become synced with circadian rhythm by around six months of age, with more time awake during the day while still frequently napping. By around age four a child has a biphasic pattern more like that of adults, but sleeping a few hours longer and napping for far longer than adults. Older, preteen children come to match the sleep pattern of adults, even as their ratio of NREM and REM is lower.

There is vastly more research and information available on sleep problems experienced by adults and the elderly than children (from infancy through adolescence), this while education and training in pediatrics and child psychology pay little attention to sleep.[3] Consequently, children's sleep problems are often treated in the same ways as those of adults, with prescription medication a common resort. Yet dating to at least Thomas Phaire's 1545 *The Boke of Chyldren,* the first pediatrics textbook, which lists "watchyng out of measure" (insomnia), "colyke and rumblying in the guttes" (infantile colic), and "pyssyng in bedde," we have known that children have some sleep problems in common with adults plus others largely unique to children. Although knowledge of children's sleep problems has increased since the beginning of the Early Modern Period in the 1500s, sleep medicine and child psychology still give short shrift to the distinctiveness of children's sleep problems, reflected in the *ICSD*'s barely polite gesture in acknowledging children's unique conditions and experiences with sleep. Yoga does no better in addressing sleep and other health conditions of children, with ancient to modern yoga literature mostly silent on children.

The special nature of children's sleep problems rests in the changes in sleep physiology during child development.[4] As mentioned earlier, infants and very young children have a far greater proportion of their sleep during REM, reflecting the intensive neural network development occurring in the young brain. An infant's circadian clock is not developed until around six months of age, causing awakenings throughout the night that can be lovingly embraced by parents, often taking turns to minimize their own sleep disturbance (well depicted by Charlize Theron in the film *Tully*). Young children continue to require more sleep than adults yet often do not get it.

Children's sleep patterns are profoundly affected by the attitudes and behaviors of their parents. Consistently loving, soothing, and comforting interaction enables a child to feel safe going to bed and falling asleep. When going to bed is a consequence of punishment, children come to associate bed with negative feelings. When going to bed occurs amid parental anger, children come to fear sleep. Considering various forms of child abuse, including sexual abuse, and exposure to domestic violence, it is not surprising that some children resist going to bed, have difficulty sleeping once in bed, and often have nightmares once asleep.[5]

Whereas adults' sleep problems tend to be chronic, those of children tend to be transient, as they are typically part of normal child development. For example, enlarged tonsils and adenoids, which can cause snoring and obstructive sleep apnea, are usually normal and self-resolve. As infants develop, they gradually gain circadian entrainment to light, leading to more regular sleep. Parents' and doctors' responses to a child's sleep issues are often a greater problem than the child's sleep issues themselves, especially in the tendency to misdiagnose or overdiagnose (e.g., assuming a child's resistance to sleep is a sign of ADHD) and thus inappropriately or prematurely resort to sleep medication.[6]

This is not to downplay the significance of sleep issues among infants, young children, and adolescents, the effects of which can affect cognitive development, cognitive function, emotional balance, physical energy, and immune system function. However, the greater tendency to make rash judgments about a child's sleep issues leads to labeling and treatments that might be unwarranted and unnecessary. In many instances, there is an underlying relational or behavioral issue, oftentimes rooted in parental behavior, that causes a child to have difficulty sleeping well.[7]

Infants

With the following insights and tips, you can help your child to develop healthy sleep habits from the time they are born:

- Remember that newborns have polyphasic sleep—their sixteen to seventeen hours per day of sleep come in short snippets during the day and night, often for only an hour or two at a time divided equally between day and night.

- In the first two years of life, nighttime sleep gradually increases from around eight or nine hours to around eleven hours, while daytime sleep gradually decreases from around eight hours to around two hours.

- By six months, most babies begin sleeping through the night, with about ten hours of nighttime sleep and about four hours of daytime sleep.

- At about six months, many babies have difficulty falling asleep or have nighttime awakenings, primarily due to separation anxiety (they do not understand that separations are temporary) or overstimulation.

- Falling asleep depends on sleepiness, which one can see in infants' yawning, rubbing their eyes, and becoming fussy. Most babies will readily fall asleep when sleepy.

- Expose your baby to sunlight in the morning and during the day, as they are developing their natural production of melatonin.

- When feeding your baby before going to sleep at night or during nighttime feedings, keep the room dimly lit and quiet, and minimize stimulation.

- You can help your baby fall asleep by putting them in their crib (not your bed) when they are sleepy yet still awake, thereby helping them to learn to fall asleep in bed.

- Follow the American Academy of Pediatrics' mantra "On Their Back, Every Nap & Every Night," placing your baby in a firm-surface crib free of pillows and blankets to reduce the risk of suffocation.

- If you are the mother's partner or helper and notice the mother dozing off with her baby on her chest, place her baby in its crib.

- From around six months, put your baby in their crib while awake and soothe him or her with soft, comforting words while sitting next to the crib, night by night moving gradually farther away from their crib.

- Do not put your baby to sleep with constant rocking or nursing.

- If your baby is crying once in their crib, allow them to cry while reassuring them for a few minutes—without picking them up.

- As infants get older, gradually decrease nap time to increase sleep pressure; do not skip naps.

- From around twelve months, give your baby a soft stuffed animal (younger infants should not be given soft objects with which to sleep due to increased risk of sudden infant death syndrome).

- Before putting your infant in the crib, devote five to ten minutes to cuddling, gazing in their eyes, softly singing, and soothing them. YouTube is filled with very sweet and precious baby sleep music that you might enjoy too.

Toddlers and Preschoolers

As every parent knows, the challenges with children's sleep can become greater as they grow out of infancy and into the fascinating time of being a toddler and very young child. Emotional factors are increasingly significant as your child gains more experience in the realm of family and other human relationships. Consider these tips to help your young child grow beyond any tendency to resist going to bed, staying in bed, and sleeping through the night.

- Teach your toddler and young children to sleep by creating the structure and interaction that make going to bed and falling asleep more natural and pleasant.

- Create a family bedtime ritual, involving your children as best as you can in shaping it.

- List and number presleep activities, and be specific, such as put away toys, put on pajamas, brush teeth, tell or read stories (how many?), sing lullabies, share cuddles (for how long? how many?), dim lights, close blinds, turn light out.

- Consider the American Academy of Pediatrics' "4 B's of Bedtime": (1) Bathing (it raises core body temperature, which helps in falling asleep); (2) Brushing (signifying no more eating); (3) Books (a wonderful way to provide loving comfort); and (4) Bedtime (a consistent time in a well-made, inviting bed).

- Stick with the plan so it becomes a regular routine, and be consistent with bedtime so there are healthier habits and fewer surprises.

- In all late-evening time together, keep the mood positive by asking about their day, telling them things that affirm your love for them (perhaps as simple as sharing something you watched them doing earlier in the day) and reinforce feeling safe going to sleep.

- Let your child bring a favorite safe toy or object to bed. This will help them feel comfortable falling asleep, and help them go back to sleep if they wake up during the night.

- Electronics should not be in any bedroom, period. (This goes for adults as well as kids.) Think of it this way: if you would not give your child a stimulating cup of coffee or soda, be consistent by not giving them a stimulating electronic device to play with before going to bed or once in bed. Both affect brain chemistry!

- Reward kids for getting to sleep and staying in bed for their full sleep opportunity, but do not reprimand them or otherwise make negative associations with sleep.

- If they get out of bed, take them back to bed while listening to what they say and responding in calm, loving ways, soothing any anxiety while being consistent with the principle of staying in bed.

- If your child is afraid, comfort them if they had a nightmare by telling them it is in their imagination and that they are safe. Provide a very dim night light, leave the door slightly open, and affirm that you are close by and will always keep them safe. Limit exposure to scary movies and images.

- If your child calls out for you, wait at least several seconds before replying and gradually wait longer each time while reassuring them you are nearby. If you go into their room, keep it dimly lit and quiet while you soothe them. Gradually stay farther from their bed when you go in, until giving reassurance without going in at all, always reminding your child that it is time to go to sleep.

- Teach your child how to relax using the breathing and postural practices given in chapter 4. Make it fun. For more ideas, explore Mariam Gates's *Good Night Yoga,* a sweet and well-informed children's book.

School-Age Children

The physiology of young children makes them naturally good sleepers. Consistency and emotional safety remain among the most important factors in healthy sleep as children begin school and expand their social circles. A new challenge arises from the disturbance of regular routines due to differing weekday and weekend schedules (as for adolescents and adults), lengthy school vacations, and the long summer holiday. Consider these insights:

- Invite your child to share with you in updating the family bedtime ritual now that they are going to school.

- Consider age-appropriate suggestions given above for toddlers and preschoolers.

- Many children experience difficulties in school due to everything from relationships with peers and adults, to learning and playground challenges. Have daily conversations with your child about his or her school day, providing emotional support and reassurance. This will help with their sleep, and better sleep helps with everything that happens at school.

- Keep the bedtime rituals simple and manageable, and try to maintain the rituals with some flexibility even on the weekends.

- Give your child nightly choices about what books to read together, what lullabies to sing, and what stuffed animal to bring to bed.

- Try to stay close to the regular bedtime schedule on weekends and holidays.

- Keep teaching your child how to relax using the breathing and postural practices given in chapter 4, always making it fun. In using Mariam Gates's *Good Night Yoga,* start inviting your child to create their own movements and postures so long as they are relaxing.

- Play with sequence 32 (for elementary school-age children) in my book *Yoga Sequencing: Designing Transformative Yoga Classes.*

Most children who do yoga come to it by mimicking their parents. Children can certainly benefit from doing yoga on a regular basis just as much as adults, developing or maintaining flexibility, strength, coordination, and balance in their bodies while reducing stress and gaining a more positive outlook on life. However, the yoga that parents do may not be appropriate for kids. It is important to take children's stage of development into consideration. Their bodies are still growing, their bones are softer, and their ligaments more elastic. Asanas that give healthy stress to the bones of an adult can overstress a child's bones. Movement that involves maximum range of motion in an adult joint can overstretch a child's ligaments, leading to long-term instability in the joint. Although it may seem that kids can run and play forever, adult yoga classes—typically an hour to an hour and a half—can cause fatigue in a child. And whereas many adults enjoy doing yoga in a highly heated room, a child doing that practice in the same room is considerably more prone to heat exhaustion.

Many simple and popular yoga postures are contraindicated in the broader literature on children's physical fitness. For example, in the California Department of Education's *Physical Education Framework for California Public Schools,* several positions that mimic or are identical to basic yoga postures are listed as contraindicated for all children in kindergarten through twelfth grade, including: Chair Pose (Utkatasana), Standing Forward Bend Pose (Uttanasana), Plow Pose (Halasana), Shoulder Stand (Salamba Sarvangasana), Extended Triangle Pose (Utthita Trikonasana), the arm position of Warrior II Pose (Virabhadrasana II), and Bound Angle Pose (Baddha Konasana, often called Butterfly Pose in children's yoga).[8] In several instances the recommended alternative appears riskier than the contraindicated position: a high lunge with the knee projected beyond the foot is the alternative to Baddha Konasana, while a slumped expression of Sage Marichi's Pose (Marichyasana A) is given as the alternative to Uttanasana.

Appreciate that most children are inherently active (unless led into a sedentary lifestyle) and that with yoga you are giving children an opportunity to direct their physical activity in specific ways to help them to develop keener awareness of being in their bodies.

Use this tips in helping your children play with yoga:

- Listen; children will teach you how to guide them.

- Appreciate that young children are inherently creative and that they will spontaneously express their creativity with the postures.

- Play with offering yoga as a form of play rather than as a disciplined practice, so that your children feel a sense of freedom in their physical exploration.

- Limit the practice to twenty-five to forty-five minutes, depending on fitness.

- Teach your children ujjayi pranayama, which is calming.

- Guide your children in feeling the movements and overall sensations in their bodies that happen with the fluctuations of the breath.

- Sprinkle the postures with stories, music, and games to more fully engage your children.

- Maximize the use of natural names for postures such as tree, frog, cat, cobra, butterfly, and so on, and encourage imaginative and expressive ways of bringing the postures more to life by "acting" these parts.

- Keep the postures simple. Be aware that as flexible as young kids are, they can easily overstretch.

- Keep the room temperature moderate and comfortable. There is absolutely no benefit to children in doing yoga in a room heated above seventy-five degrees Fahrenheit.

- Appreciate that children are different from one another and can benefit from sequences that address their uniqueness.

- In working with hyperactive children, help to channel their energy by offering sequences that involve movement. Standing and balancing asanas are an excellent way for these children to direct their more impulsive energy in healthy ways.

- Use creative visualization in Savasana (Corpse Pose, which you can call "Resting Pose") to encourage relaxation. Read a short story during their Savasana.

Adolescents

A significant change in sleep timing occurs in adolescence with a shift in circadian rhythm. With the advent of puberty, the timing of our suprachiasmatic nucleus moves forward, regardless of geography, culture, and parental expectations, making it increasingly natural to go to sleep a few hours later and to sleep a few hours later in the morning.[9] Adolescents also spend a greater amount of time in NREM sleep as their brains are pruning the neural architecture for more efficient and effective performance, making it more difficult to rouse them from sleep and giving them the highest sleep efficiency of any age. This pattern is present from puberty until around age twenty-two.

Asking your fifteen-year-old to go to sleep before 11 p.m. and wake up eight hours later goes directly against what is happening with their body chemistry. Healthy adolescent development, including learning in school, is undermined by forcing teenagers to sleep, wake, and learn on a schedule designed for parental and institutional needs in modern society (with school schedules fashioned around the needs of businesses, government agencies, and those who work in them). Consequently, 80 percent of adolescents get less than the nine hours of sleep per night they need for healthy development and functioning, a problem compounded by the ill-informed expectation that teenagers are ready for sleep when their parents are (or earlier), this despite the shift in adolescent circadian rhythm toward being sleepy about three hours later than adults. This has significant deleterious effects on school performance, social skills, and emotional balance.

There are many factors that exacerbate adolescent sleep and health problems. Many adolescents struggle with matters of personal identity, individuation, sexuality, interpersonal and social relationships, violence, and academic pressure. Poor diet, lack of healthy exercise, obesity, eating disorders, drug abuse, smoking, and the consequences (or potential consequences) of risky behavior further contribute to worries, anxiety, and depression, which in turn are frequently given as reasons for sleep problems during adolescence. This array of factors also makes suicide the second leading cause of death at this age (with soaring rates across the United States in recent years).[10]

Not surprisingly, conventional medical and psychiatric approaches to adolescent sleep problems typically prescribe behavior modification, chronotherapy (the use of bright light to change the timing of the sleep phase), and medication, this rather than honoring changes in adolescent physiology and modifying the institutional schedules that otherwise exacerbate the effects of these changes.[11] A recent upsurge in research on the often complex etiology and associations of adolescent sleep problems is stimulating greater subtlety in both understanding and treatment.[12] More humanistic and enlightened approaches are changing school start times, with evidence showing that better sleep reduces risky behaviors, the incidence of depression, and teenage car crashes (the leading cause of teenage deaths in the United States) while enhancing student academic achievement.[13] While the suggestions for better adolescent sleep offered here focus on sleep hygiene and yoga, concerned parents might fruitfully work with their local and regional school agencies to change school start times in order to accommodate teenagers' natural sleep needs.

Notwithstanding teenagers' sleep phase delay, it is important to engage teenagers in ways that bring them to make healthy sleep a high priority in their lives. As with younger children, adolescents tend to sleep longer on the weekends, complicating their sleep problems during the week. Even if sleeping less than nine hours per night, it is important to be consistent in sleep-wake times. It is also important to cut out caffeine late in the day, whether from so-called energy drinks, sodas, coffee, tea, or chocolate. It is equally important to cut out exposure to LED screens (phones, tablets, computers) within one to two hours of going to bed. And like younger children and adults, adolescents need a bedroom that is their sleep haven—quiet, dark, cool, and comfortable.

Yoga for Better Adolescent Sleep

If you are a young adolescent, review the guidelines for school-age children, then move forward from there depending on how you feel with the postures. For all adolescents, appreciate the larger conditions of your life, considering tendencies toward hyperarousal, lethargy, and depression, then refer to chapters 4–6 for appropriate practices. Limit your practices to forty-five to sixty minutes, depending on fitness, while recognizing that many teens enjoy taking regular yoga classes that are as long as ninety minutes.

For adolescents with sleep problems, practice yoga early in the day, or if in the evening, practice at least two hours before going to bed. Some yoga studios offer yoga classes designed for teenagers, yet often these classes are similar to adult classes except being for shorter duration. Try to find classes that allow creativity, that are playful, yet that at the same time invite you to explore self-awareness and self-discipline. Remember that many teens are chronically tired due to inadequate sleep; at first, you might not seem motivated, but once the class starts most teens get interested.

Due to being tired and for emotional reasons, many teens (like many adults) have slouched posture that is unhealthy for the spine and inhibits breathing. It is important to have yoga classes that emphasize stable grounding, which is the foundation for establishing the natural and neutral form of the spine. Do the basic yoga breathing technique of ujjayi pranayama, exploring how in breathing deeply you can more easily support your healthy posture.

Play around with appropriately challenging postures. In doing so, be aware that your body is still developing and it is not healthy for you to go into extreme ranges of motion or hold complex postures for long periods of time. To help counter the effects of slouched postures, teen classes ideally have easy backbends such as Bridge Pose (Setu Bandha Sarvangasana), which are mildly stimulating. After backbends, simple twists help reduce tension along the spine, and forward bends help in calming down in the later phase of a class. With teens who are hyperactive, hyperaroused, or overstimulated, doing Savasana (Corpse Pose) for five to seven minutes can be greatly calming.

Although many teens (and adults) react to the idea of meditation with distaste (less and less as yoga and mindfulness practices further enter the cultural mainstream), most teens are open to it when it is demystified and its potential fruits highlighted. Appreciate that meditation is not about having a perfectly quiet mind, but rather about allowing the mind to settle and coming into more calm and clear awareness. The meditation practices in chapters 4–6 are appropriate for you.

Enjoy exploring yoga, knowing it will help you with your sleep and energy!

Older Adults

From middle age on, our sleep architecture and sleep patterns gradually change.[14] Later in life, we encounter other changes in our sleep tendencies, such as the hot flashes of menopause and the weakening bladder and slightly regressed circadian rhythm of older age. The circadian rhythm in older adults moves the opposite way we find with adolescents, causing the slow-wave deep sleep of adolescence to fade further and further away as the rhythm is less and less synchronized with natural light patterns, with natural sleep onset occurring earlier in the evening.[15] If an elderly person intermittently dozes in accordance with their circadian clock instead of going to sleep for the night, their sleep pressure drops and they tend to have more fragmented sleep. This leads to a greater tendency to nap the next day, more dozing in the evening, and a growing problem getting healthy sleep.

Deep sleep is increasingly elusive as we move beyond middle age, with REM sleep decreasing as our circadian rhythm is desynchronized (the SCN is deteriorating, natural melatonin secretion is decreasing, and exposure to light tends to diminish).[16] In older age, sleep onset occurs earlier in the evening, with subsequent waking that much earlier in the morning. Even though in bed for longer periods of time, the elderly experience less sleep efficiency and less total time asleep.[17]

These tendencies toward fragmented, lighter, and less sleep in older adults are exacerbated by several factors. Women often experience insomnia from some of the effects of menopause, including hot flashes, night sweats, and depression.[18] Due to prostate enlargement, older men tend to have increasing nocturia, frequently awakening during the night to urinate, with their sleep fragmentation associated with diminished motor skills. Arthritis, respiratory difficulties, heart problems, and dementing diseases—Alzheimer's, Parkinson's, Lewy body, and other neurological changes—can lead to greater difficulty falling asleep and staying asleep.[19] Depression and anxiety arising from these conditions and one's larger (and longer) life can worsen sleep problems, while fragmented and reduced time asleep make depression and anxiety more likely and worse.[20] The medications prescribed for treating these conditions and other health conditions, ranging from beta blockers and bronchodilators to diuretics and psychiatric drugs, can all contribute to further sleep disturbance. With greater sleep disturbance, there is diminished cognitive function and motor skills, which, given the greater risk of falling and breaking increasingly brittle bones, can be especially problematic.[21]

Amid these conditions of sleep disturbance among the elderly, we find three primary sleep disorders: (1) sleep-disordered breathing (from snoring to sleep apnea); (2) periodic limb movement and, related, restless legs syndrome; and (3) REM sleep behavior disorder in which muscle atonia is attenuated, causing the appearance of acting out one's dreams.[22] These disorders are typically treated much the same as we find with younger people, with appliances for sleep-disordered breathing and medication for movement-related disorders.

The conventional treatment of circadian rhythm changes and insomnia in older adults (which are related yet often distinct, pointing to the importance of nuanced assessment and treatment) is basically the same as for younger adults, with CBT and medications leading the way. Sleep hygiene is—and should be—followed as best as possible, including reducing alcohol intake, which is particularly problematic for older adults, as this adds a second factor contributing to sleep fragmentation, earlier awakening, and the risk of falling when walking to the bathroom during the night. In contrast to younger people with either circadian rhythm disturbance (including from jet lag or shift work) or insomnia, the phase advance in the elderly to earlier sleep onset and earlier awakening points to the importance of the elderly having greater exposure to natural and bright light in the late afternoon and evening while minimizing exposure to bright light in the morning.[23]

Yoga for Better Sleep in Older Adults

Depending on your overall fitness and health conditions, the practices offered in chapters 4–6 are appropriate for older adults. Explore them! If you are an older adult with a breathing-related sleep disorder, see chapter 8 for guidance. If you are an older adult with very limited mobility, frailty, or difficulty with balance, see chapter 9 for more accessible yoga postures that are done with a standard chair. If you have osteoarthritis, be aware of pressure in your joints and back away from any sharp pain. If you have advanced osteoporosis, do not do spinal forward bends, as they can cause serious injury to your spine. As with everyone, make the breath the heart of your yoga practice, exploring the breath as an insightful barometer indicating how far to go.

Chapter

8

YOGA SEQUENCE FOR SLEEP APNEA

Sleep Apnea

Sleep apnea, often associated with snoring, is the most common type of sleep-related breathing disorder. Central sleep apnea (CSA), in which the brain fails to control respiration, is found among about 1 percent of adults aged forty and older.[1] There is no evidence that yoga can directly help. In contrast, with obstructive sleep apnea (OSA), found among about 7 percent of the general population (primarily in overweight men over age forty), yoga can help.

The medical approach to sleep apnea focuses primarily on management rather than treatment. The most common management tool is a continuous positive airway pressure (CPAP) device that uses pressurized air to forcefully maintain the opening of the airway. Nasal, pharyngeal, and other types of obstruction are often addressed with surgery. Other management tools include neurostimulation, medication, the CPAP device, and a variety of other oral appliances. Sleep position is often addressed but difficult to manage.[2] Sleep and respiratory medical professionals also encourage weight loss and exercise, which are found to reduce the incidence of mild and moderate OSA.[3]

Yoga Sequence for Sleep Apnea

Here we focus on three strategies to help with sleep apnea: reducing weight, restoring the tongue's essential role in healthy respiration using tongue/mouth exercises, and developing respiratory strength and capacity.

Step 1: Weight Loss Practices

Exercise and weight loss (if overweight) are essential tools in potentially helping with sleep apnea.[4] We cannot say that yoga generally helps to reduce weight except insofar as doing yoga brings about greater awareness of overall lifestyle, including what, when, how, and how much we eat. Rather, yoga helps to balance your overall health, including metabolic processes and digestion, thereby causing healthier weight. In doing yoga, some people gain weight, while others lose weight.

An important factor affecting yoga and weight is the type of yoga one is doing, how one is doing it, and how often. If your physical condition allows you to do vigorous exercise, yoga practices such as Vinyasa flow, Ashtanga Vinyasa, or Bikram might help you burn calories. Many other physical conditions indicate doing gentler types of yoga in which few calories are burned. Therefore, if you are unable to do vigorous yoga, you can explore other means of weight loss such as reducing caloric intake and finding other ways to burn calories, such as riding an exercise bike or walking. If this is your condition, I recommend doing the "Basic Yoga Sleep Sequence" (chapter 4) in the evening after exercising earlier in the day in a way that maximizes the burning of calories.

Step 2: Tongue and Mouth Exercises

The tongue plays an important role in respiration, although with aging it is less effective, making swallowing and breathing more difficult.[5] There is significant evidence that tongue and mouth exercises can strengthen the tongue (which is a muscle).[6] There is also evidence that a stronger, more toned, and more easily controlled tongue helps with breathing.[7] There are a variety of tongue and mouth exercises; developed primarily for use in speech therapy, some are akin to tongue, mouth, and throat exercises done in yoga, specifically the *talavya kriya, jalandhara bandha,* and *simhasana* practices presented here. We will adapt these practices to better serve healthy breathing, including with progressive resistance tongue exercises.

Talavya Kriya

Described in the fifteenth-century *Hatha Yoga Pradipika* as "milking" the tongue, in *talavya kriya* (from *talavya,* "palate" or "mouth") we stretch and massage the tongue.[8] This practice is offered as preparation for *khechari mudra,* in which the frenulum linguae under the tongue is gradually stretched and cut away to allow the tongue to draw back and up into the nasal passages, where it is said to receive the nectar of the divine—*amrita* ("immortality").

1. Brush your teeth, scrape your tongue with a tongue scraper, then rinse your mouth.

2. Using a clean white cotton towel, thoroughly rub the insides of your cheeks and the roof of your mouth.

3. Using a clean part of the towel, clasp your tongue.

4. Very gently pull your tongue forward as far as you comfortably can, and hold it in this stretched position for up to ten seconds while breathing steadily. Relax for several breaths, then repeat up to five times.

5. Gently pull your tongue to the right and hold for ten seconds. Switch sides. Relax for several breaths, then repeat up to five times.

6. Twist your tongue as far in one direction as you comfortably can, and hold for ten seconds. Switch directions. Relax for several breaths, then repeat up to five times.

7. Alternate squeezing your tongue from top to bottom and side to side for up to one minute.

8. Putting the towel aside, open your mouth and draw the tip of your tongue up and toward the back of the roof of your mouth, then slide it toward the back of your teeth, going back and forth ten times. With your tongue pressed back, hold for ten seconds. Relax for several breaths, then repeat up to five times.

9. Stick your tongue out as far as you can and hold for ten seconds. Relax for several breaths, then repeat up to five times.

10. Press the tip of your tongue firmly into the inside of your right cheek and hold for ten seconds. Switch sides. Relax for several breaths, then repeat up to five times.

11. Press the tip of your tongue against the back of your upper teeth and hold for ten seconds. Relax for several breaths, then repeat up to five times.

12. Stick your tongue out as far as you can and press it firmly against a clean spoon. Maintaining firm pressure against the spoon, slowly retract and prolapse your tongue ten times. Relax for several breaths, then repeat up to five times.

Jalandhara Bandha

Traditionally taught as a mechanism for retaining amrita, *jalandhara bandha* (from *jal,* "throat," and *bandha,* "to bind") can help in strengthening the suprahyoid muscles that assist in elevating the hyoid bone, which is located directly beneath the tongue. Lifting the hyoid bone is an important part of swallowing; weakness in these muscles disturbs swallowing and breathing.[9] The practice given here combines jalandhara bandha with modern techniques for strengthening the suprahyoid muscles.

1. Sitting comfortably tall with your shoulder blades relaxed down your back, place your hands on your knees.

2. Do several cycles of ujjayi pranayama, focusing on steadiness and ease in the flow of the breath.

3. Inhaling as deeply as you comfortably can, hold the breath.

4. Bring your chin slightly forward, slightly down, then in toward your collarbones.

5. Pressing your hands down onto your knees, lift your shoulders (sensitive to your neck).

6. Hold for up to thirty seconds, then raise your head back to the neutral starting position and slowly release the breath.

7. Repeat five to ten times.

8. Next, open your mouth as wide as you can and hold it open for fifteen seconds. Relax for several breaths, then repeat up to five times.

Simhasana

Simhasana (Lion Pose) is both a posture and breathing technique. It is traditionally taught sitting on the heels with the ankles crossed. To make this more accessible, consider sitting in a comfortable cross-legged position (consider sitting on a bolster or in a chair if necessary for stability and ease).

1. Place your palms firmly down on your knees with your fingers spread apart like the claws of a lion.

2. Inhaling through your nose, slightly lift your chin.

3. With a smooth yet strong exhalation through your mouth, stretch the tip of your tongue toward your chin and gaze upward while creating a strong "haaaa" sound as the breath flows out.

4. Repeat five to ten times.

Step 3: Respiratory Strengthening

Because poor breathing and weak respiratory function are frequently found in those with sleep apnea, it is important to go deeper in creating potentially effective treatments to help with sleep apnea. Respiratory strength training can help.[10] Here we suggest trying several breathing practices that help in developing greater respiratory strength and capacity.

Kumbhaka Pranayama

Kumbhaka is the practice of staying with and expanding the natural pause between inhalations and exhalations. In holding the breath in these pauses, the bodymind becomes more still and clear. There are two forms: *antara kumbhaka* is retention of the inhalation; *bahya kumbhaka* is retention of the exhalation. It is important to develop these practices slowly, gradually refining the neuromuscular intelligence of the diaphragm, intercostal muscles, and other secondary respiratory muscles. This practice should not cause any strain. Take it easy in expanding the duration of retention.

Antara Kumbhaka

1. Sitting in a comfortable upright position, come into natural breathing.

2. Begin to cultivate ujjayi pranayama, the gradual deepening of the breath. The spine should be naturally erect and relaxed, the heart center spacious and soft, the brain as light and quiet as possible in that moment.

3. Using the basic breath awareness practices discussed earlier, focus your attention on the natural pause at the crest of the inhalations, noticing what happens in your body-mind and larger sense of being in that space.

4. Allow a feeling of seamless movement into and out of the pause, staying with this simple practice for several rounds of breath.

5. Explore antara kumbhaka, retaining the inhalations for a few seconds.

6. Hold the breath with as little effort as possible while tuning in to the shifting sensations in your body and mental awareness.

7. In transitioning into the exhalation, the tendency is for the breath to rush out; if that happens, try a shorter duration of retention.

8. After one antara kumbhaka, do several rounds of ujjayi pranayama, restoring the lungs to their natural condition. The rhythm of inhalation and exhalation should

be smooth and steady before doing further antara kumbhaka.

9. Next, gradually lengthen the duration of retention, but only so far as there is no strain, imbalance in inhalations and exhalations, or gripping or collapsing in the lungs.

10. Explore expanding the retention by one or two counts in each sitting, eventually holding the breath in as long as you can with complete comfort.

Bahya Kumbhaka

1. Begin bahya kumbhaka after you are at ease doing antara kumbhaka.

2. Start with ujjayi pranayama, bringing attention to the natural pause when empty of breath. Do several rounds of ujjayi pranayama, refining awareness of the movement in and out of that pause.

3. With the first few retentions of the exhalation, hold for just one count and then do several rounds of seamless ujjayi pranayama before repeating.

4. Gradually expand the count, staying with simple retention. Try to keep your eyes, face, throat, and heart center soft and not to grip in your belly.

5. To release bahya kumbhaka, it is important first to completely relax the belly and thereby allow the diaphragm to do its natural work; then consciously ease the breath in.

6. If the breath rushes in, it was held in bahya kumbhaka for too long.

7. Gradually develop this practice by lengthening the duration of retention and by adding antara kumbhaka in the same rounds of breath.

8. Gradually work toward doing the kumbhaka practice for three to five minutes, stretching everything—the length of the inhalation, exhalation, and retentions.

Sama and Visama Vrtti Pranayama

1. Sitting comfortably, start to breathe with an ujjayi pranayama quality.

2. Cultivate the breath by making your breathing as steady and calm, yet as spacious, as you can comfortably sustain (sthira sukham pranayama).

3. After the completion of each inhalation and exhalation, allow the natural momentary pause that happens in the movement of the breath. That moment of stillness is a sign and source of being relaxed and present in what you are doing.

4. Cultivating *sama vrtti* ("same fluctuation"), make your inhalations and exhalations more alike in pace, duration, and the texture of the breath. Breathe this way for ten cycles of breath.

5. Explore lengthening your inhalation by a count of one or two, creating *visama vrtti* ("unequal fluctuation"). In stretching the length of the inhalation, do so only so much that the following exhalation does not rush out and such that there is no disturbance to steadiness and ease. Breathe this way for ten cycles of breath.

6. Come back to sama vrtti, resuming the initial length of your inhalations and exhalations for a few cycles of breath.

7. Now explore lengthening your exhalation by a count of one or two, again creating visama vrtti. In stretching the

length of the exhalation, do so only so much that the following inhalation does not rush out and such that there is no disturbance to steadiness and ease. Breathe this way for ten cycles of breath.

8. Maintaining the stretched length of your exhalations, lengthen your inhalations to match your exhalations, breathing more deeply in and more fully out for one to two minutes.

9. Come back to natural breathing and relax.

10. Doing this practice daily, explore gradually lengthening your inhalations and exhalations a little more in each session.

Viloma Pranayama

The term *viloma,* which in literal translation means "anti-hair," refers to going against the natural line or movement of the breath. In *viloma pranayama,* one repeatedly pauses during the inhalation and exhalation while changing as little as possible in the positioning and engagement of the diaphragm, rib cage, and lungs. With practice, our awareness is steady throughout each cycle of breath, the nerves calm and quiet in support of both flow and pause.

Begin by sitting up comfortably tall, and do several rounds of ujjayi pranayama, focusing on the balance and ease in the breath, then explore as follows:

1. After a complete exhalation, inhale to half your capacity and hold the breath there for a few seconds before completing the inhalation.

2. Repeat several times before adding a second interruption to the inhalation, continuing in this way until you reach five pauses, and only so long as there is no strain or fatigue.

3. Follow this with several rounds of ujjayi pranayama before resting in Savasana.

4. Next, repeat this exercise with pauses in the exhalations only.

5. When the lungs are empty, let the diaphragm relax and the belly draw farther back and up before easing into the inhalation.

6. After resting in Savasana for a few minutes, do viloma pranayama on both the inhalation and exhalation.

7. If you are free of strain in doing viloma, begin doing kumbhakas along with it, as follows.

8. Start with antara kumbhaka following a viloma pranayama inhalation in which there are one or more interruptions, keeping the diaphragm soft during the pauses.

9. With the antara kumbhaka, retain the inhalation for two or three seconds before exhaling, gradually holding for longer.

10. After gradually developing this practice for up to ten minutes in each sitting, do viloma pranayama exhalations as described earlier, followed by bahya kumbhaka, gradually increasing the viloma interruptions and the length of bahya kumbhaka.

11. For the full practice of viloma pranayama, explore viloma inhalations and exhalations along with antara and bahya kumbhaka, slowly lengthening the practice.

Nadi Shodhana Pranayama

This practice is said to harmonize the hemispheres of the brain. It is also helpful in developing respiratory capacity.

1. Sit comfortably and practice ujjayi pranayama for a few minutes.

2. Place the fingertips on one side of the nose, the thumb on the other side, just below the slight notch about half-way down the side of the nose. Try to place the fingers with even pressure on the left and right sides of the nose, maintaining steady contact while keeping the nostrils fully open.

3. While continuing ujjayi pranayama, play with slightly varying the pressure of the fingers, becoming more sensitive to the effects of the fine finger adjustments.

4. After a complete exhalation, close the right nostril and slowly inhale through the left.

5. At the crest of the inhalation, close the left nostril and slowly exhale through the right.

6. Empty of breath, fully inhale through the right, close the right, and exhale through the left.

7. Continue with this initial form of alternate nostril breathing for up to five minutes, cultivating the smooth and steady flow of the breath while remaining relaxed and calm.

8. Repeat this practice daily.

9. To go further, explore bringing the viloma and kumbhaka practices into your nadi shodhana practice.

Chapter 9

CHAIR YOGA FOR BETTER SLEEP

Introduction: Sitting Down to Sit Up

Most yoga postures are not accessible to those with significant mobility, balance, or frailty issues. Yet many yoga postures can be done using a stable chair or lying on the floor. Doing yoga with a chair enables even strong and healthy people to hold postures longer and to be more comfortable doing yoga breathing and meditation practices. Although it is ideal to practice yoga free of a chair, this simple prop opens the practice to a wide range of people with challenging conditions ranging from chronic pain and carpal tunnel syndrome to osteoporosis and multiple sclerosis.

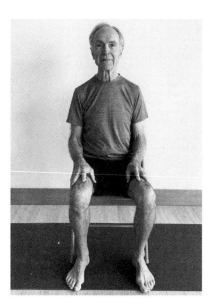

The ideal chair for yoga is a folding metal chair. It is stable, provides a firm foundation, and can be easily clasped for self-assistance in many postures. A few of the postures described in the following sequence are done on the floor with the support or assistance of other props. The postures done with the chair can be equally well explored sitting in an office chair or on a plane or train.

Choosing a Sequence

There are optional choices you can make in what follows in keeping with your conditions and intentions. For the basic practice, read the introduction to chapter 4. If you tend to be anxious or hyperaroused, read the introduction to chapter 5. If you tend to be depressed or lethargic, read the introduction to chapter 6. With each of these conditions, note the recommendations regarding special sensitivity for each posture.

What You Will Need

- A stable chair, blankets or bolsters, strap, block

Doing the Sequence

Step 1: Sitting and Breathing

Getting Situated: Sitting on your chair, place your feet on the floor hip-distance apart. If you are unable to press your feet firmly into the floor, elevate your feet onto blocks (large books serve this purpose well). Try to position your pelvis with your weight toward the front of your sitting bones. If unable to do this, use a folded blanket to elevate your sitting bones. Rooting firmly down into your sitting bones, try to sit as comfortably tall as you can without using the back of the chair for support.

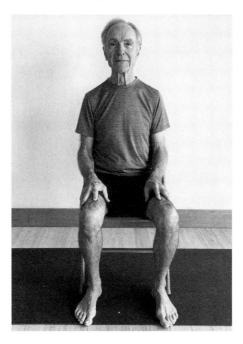

Tuning In: Let your eyes rest lightly closed, or, alternatively, softly focus your gaze on a point nearby. Bring your awareness to your breathing, simply noticing it, feeling it, and being with it. Sense the breath flowing in and out, and how your body is moving with the breath. Notice if you are doing anything that disturbs the simple flow of the breath. With the completion of each inhalation and exhalation, notice the slight pause, a momentary suspension, in the movement of the breath. Try always to allow these natural pauses to happen. Allow the breath to flow as freely and easily as you can for about one to two minutes.

Ujjayi Pranayama: Changing as little as possible in your comfort and the flow of the breath, open your mouth and breathe out as though you are trying to breathe fog onto a glass or mirror. In doing so, sense the breath in your throat and how when it flows over your vocal cords it gives the breath a light whisper-like sound. Maintain this sound and sensation of the breath in your throat as you draw the breath in. Do this for three cycles of breath. Now keep breathing with this sound and sensation but with your mouth closed, using the sensations of the breath to make it smoother and simpler. Breathe with this ujjayi—uplifting—technique when doing any yoga posture, including when transitioning in and out of the postures.

Sama and Visama Vrtti Pranayama: In sama and visama vrtti breathing, make the pace and duration of the breath equal (sama) or unequal (visama) as it flows (vrtti). Start with sama vrtti, with an ujjayi quality. Cultivate the breath by making your breathing as steady and calm, yet as spacious, as you can comfortably sustain (sthira sukham pranayama). Whenever doing yoga postures, try to establish sama vrtti with ujjayi as the default. Then, to more deeply relax and release tension, explore stretching the length of each exhalation by a count of one or two, thus breathing with unequal fluctuation (visama vrtti). In stretching the length of the exhalation, do so only so much that the following inhalation does not rush in and such that there is no disturbance to sthira sukham pranayama.

Breathe in this way for three to five minutes. With each inhalation, enjoy the simple and light ways your body naturally expands. Allow the natural pause that happens when filled with breath. With the breath flowing out, sense the natural ways your body settles, especially as you stretch the length of the exhalations a little more. As this settling happens, allow your body to relax a little more deeply. With every inhalation, feel where you sense tension in your body or your thoughts. With every exhalation, let go.

In preparation for step 2, come up to standing, shake out your legs, and then come back to sitting on the chair.

Step 2: Yoga Postures in a Chair

Note: In doing any of the following postures in which you are sitting with both sitting bones on the chair, begin with the directions for sitting and breathing given in step 1.

Special Sensitivities:

- If you have arthritis, be gentle in your movements to minimize pain in your joints.

- If you have advanced osteoporosis, be especially sensitive to pressure in your spine and do not fold forward through your torso (i.e., minimize spinal flexion).

- If you have had a hip replacement with posterior entry, do not flex your hip beyond ninety degrees, do not cross the leg of the hip replacement over the other leg (i.e., do not adduct it), and avoid strong internal rotation of the hip (as happens when walking pigeon-toed). With anterior-entry hip replacement, do not do deep lunges in which the leg of the hip that was operated on is extended back from the hip).

Sufi Circles

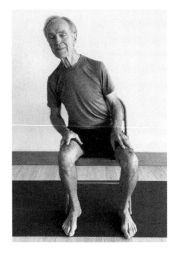 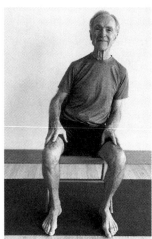

Special Sensitivity: Low back, neck, knees, shoulders
Props: Chair, possibly blocks and a blanket
Doing the Pose: Slowly move your spine circularly in one direction for one minute, gradually expanding the circles while breathing deeply, then go the other direction for one minute. Try to keep your sitting bones firmly rooted, and maintain a comfortably upright posture amid these movements.

Cat-Cow

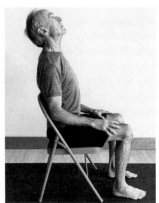

Special Sensitivity: Low back, neck, knees, shoulders. Cat position is contraindicated if you have advanced osteoporosis.
Props: Chair, possibly blocks and a blanket
Doing the Pose: While breathing deeply in, extend taller through your spine. As you release the breath, slowly arch your spine into the Cat position.

With the next inhalation, arch your spine forward into the Cow position. Continue these movements for one to two minutes.

Twist

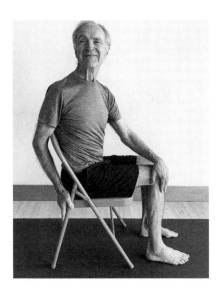

Special Sensitivity: Low back, neck, knees, shoulders
Props: Chair, possibly blocks and a blanket
Doing the Pose: Place your right hand on your left knee, and clasp the side or seat of the chair with your left hand. Let your shoulder blades release down your back to allow more ease through your neck. While inhaling, lightly pull up with your left hand to help draw yourself more upright through your spine. As you exhale, lightly press your right hand against your left knee to encourage the twist. With each successive inhalation slightly back away from the twist to again lift taller through your spine, and with each successive exhalation explore twisting farther to the left. Try to create the twist from your lower sternum, adding movement in your low back and neck last. Continue for five to ten breaths, then switch directions.

Side Stretch

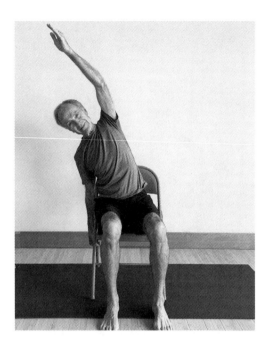

Special Sensitivity: Low back, neck, knees, shoulders. Be especially sensitive to an unstable shoulder (weak rotator cuff), frozen shoulder, impingement syndrome, and thoracic outlet syndrome.

Props: Chair, possibly blocks and a blanket

Doing the Pose: Place your right hand on the chair next to your right hip. Release your left arm down by your side, stretching from your shoulder to your fingertips. Rotate your upper arm back to turn your palm outward (external rotation of the shoulder). Slowly reach your arm out to the left, if possible until overhead. Use your right hand for stability as you explore stretching your left arm more overhead and arching over to the right. When at your maximum comfortable stretch, hold for five breaths. Switch sides.

Shoulder Rolls

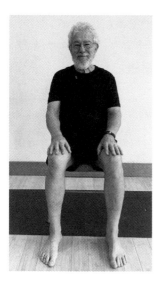

Special Sensitivity: Low back, neck, knees, shoulders

Props: Chair, possibly blocks and a blanket

Doing the Pose: Place your hands on your knees. Inhaling, draw your shoulders forward, up, and toward your ears. Exhaling, draw your shoulders back and down to the neutral starting position. Continue for thirty seconds, then switch directions, moving your shoulders back, up, forward, and down.

Eagle Arms

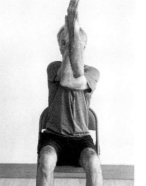

Special Sensitivity: Shoulders

Props: Chair, possibly blocks and a blanket

Doing the Pose: Extend your arms forward from your shoulders and turn your palms to face each other. Cross your right elbow over your left elbow. If unable to fully cross your elbows, use your left hand to pull your right arm across your chest. If you have your elbows fully crossed, rotate your forearms up and try to clasp your right thumb with your left hand or, going farther, try to bring your palms together. Keeping your elbows level with your shoulders, squeeze them together while pressing your hands away from your face. With each inhalation, slightly lift your chin. With each exhalation, gently draw your chin toward your chest. Continue for up to one minute.

Chest and Shoulder Stretch

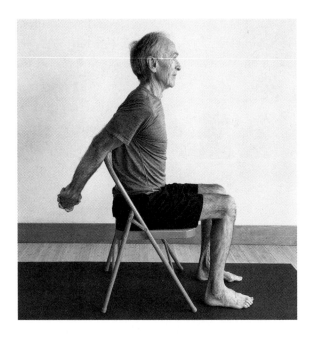

Special Sensitivity: Front of your shoulders, neck

Props: Chair, possibly a strap, blocks, and a blanket

Doing the Pose: Sit ninety degrees to the side on your chair so there is space behind you to lift your arms. Interlace your fingers behind your back. If unable to comfortably and fully interlace your fingers behind your back without straining or hunching forward, clasp a strap behind your back with your hands shoulder-distance apart or wider. With each inhalation, lift your sternum. With each exhalation, try to keep your sternum lifted while lifting your arms up away from your back. Hold for one to two minutes.

Sun Salutations

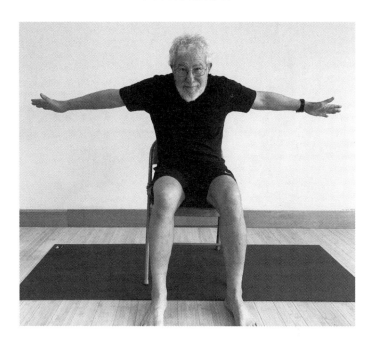

Special Sensitivity: Shoulders, low back, neck. Do this movement in the morning, in the afternoon, or when you feel prematurely sleepy in the early evening.

Props: Chair, possibly blocks and a blanket

Doing the Pose: Stretch your arms down by your sides and turn your palms outward. With each inhalation, slowly reach your arms outward and up overhead. With each exhalation, swan dive forward only as far as it is comfortable in your low back. With each successive inhalation, swan dive back up with your arms reaching overhead. Continue for up to one minute.

Knee Extensions

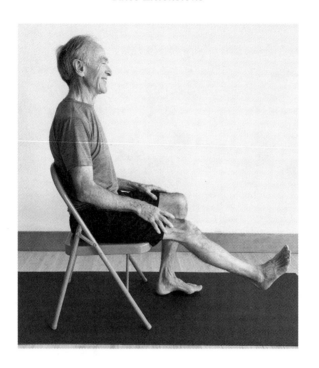

Special Sensitivity: Hamstrings, knees, low back

Props: Chair, possibly blocks and a blanket

Doing the Pose: While committing to keeping your pelvis level (neutral) and your spine in its natural shape, with each inhalation slowly lift your foot up to extend your leg straight. With each exhalation, slowly release your foot back down. Repeat five to ten times. The last time you extend your leg, try to keep it extended for five to ten breaths. Switch sides.

Leg Lifts

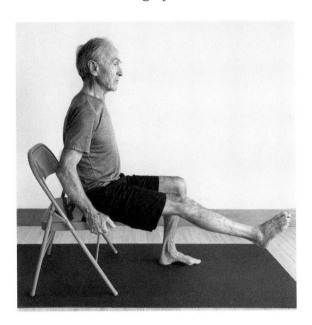

Special Sensitivity: Hamstrings, knees, low back

Props: Chair, possibly blocks and a blanket

Doing the Pose: Slide forward on the chair seat until your sitting bones are close to the edge while still stable (and no risk of tipping forward off the chair). Keep your pelvis level (neutral) and your spine in its natural shape. Stretch both legs straight, keeping your heels on the floor. With each inhalation, slowly lift your right leg up as high as you comfortably can with your low back rounded. With each exhalation, slowly release your leg down. Repeat five to ten times, then switch sides.

Goddess

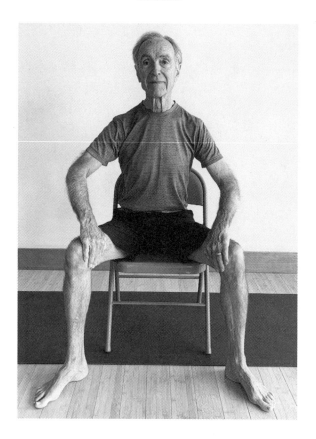

Special Sensitivity: Inner thighs and knees
Props: Chair, possibly blocks and a blanket
Doing the Pose: Place your feet wide apart and turn them out about forty-five degrees such that your knees are aligned with the centers of your feet. Place your hands on your inner thighs to press your knees farther away from each other. When at your maximum comfortable stretch, hold for one minute.

Warrior II to Extended Side-Angle Pose

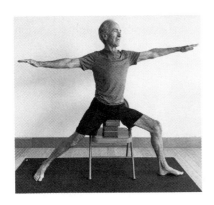 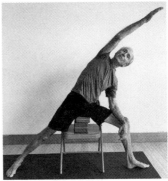

Special Sensitivity: Knees, spine (especially low back and neck), ribs, shoulders. These postures are mildly stimulating; if hyperaroused, do not do them in the evening.

Props: Chair, possibly blocks and a blanket

Doing the Pose: Beginning with Warrior II, rotate your left leg out from the hip to point your left knee ninety degrees to the left, aligning your left knee directly above the ankle. Stretch your right leg to the right, pointing it the opposite direction from your left leg and extending it as straight as you can. Try to keep both feet evenly placed on the floor and actively rooted down. Place your hands on your inner thighs to press them back. Rooting your sitting bones and drawing upright through your torso, reach your arms out over your legs and level with the floor with your palms facing down. Keeping your shoulder blades rooted down against your back ribs, stretch from the middle of your upper back and chest out through your arms and fingertips. Hold for five breaths. Transitioning to Extended Side-Angle Pose, reach out through your left arm and place your left elbow on your left knee. Turn your right hand up, then slowly stretch your right arm over your right ear. Hold for five breaths while stretching from your rooted right foot through your right fingertips.

Lunge

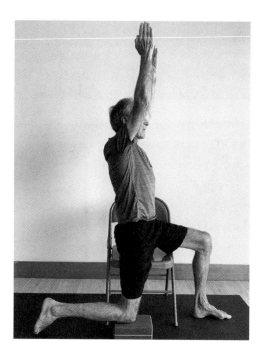

Special Sensitivity: Knees, low back. Back leg position is contraindicated if you have had an anterior-entry hip replacement.

Props: Chair, possibly blocks and a blanket, possibly a wall, a table, or an additional chair

Doing the Pose: Turn ninety degrees to your left, keeping your left sitting bone on the chair seat with your right knee toward the floor. Consider using a wall, a table, or an additional chair for your right hand in maintaining balance on the chair. Inhaling, lift tall through your torso. Without leaning your torso forward, while exhaling slide your right foot back. While inhaling slide the foot forward; while exhaling slide it back. Repeat five times, then hold for five breaths while pressing your right leg back. Switch sides.

Bridge

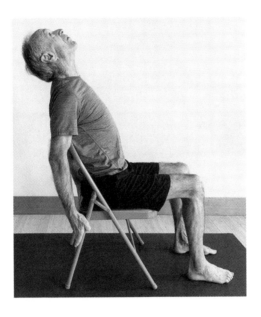

Special Sensitivity: Low back, neck, shoulders
Props: Chair, possibly blocks and a blanket
Doing the Pose: Interlace your fingers behind the back of the chair. If unable to comfortably and fully interlace your fingers behind your back without straining or hunching forward, clasp a strap behind your back with your hands shoulder-distance apart or wider. Keeping your chin drawn slightly down toward your chest, with each inhalation lift your chest while stretching your arms back away from your back. Sensitive to your neck, explore gradually lifting your chin, slowly creating a deeper arch through your spine. Hold for five to ten breaths. If depressed or

lethargic, repeat two to three times. After this posture, repeat the twist described earlier in this sequence.

Wide-Leg Forward Fold

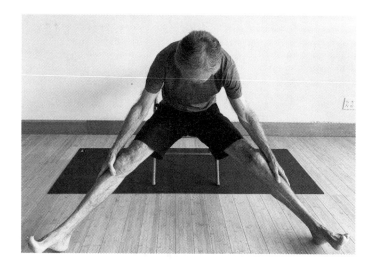

Special Sensitivity: Hamstrings, inner thighs, low back

Props: Chair, possibly a blanket, and a wall, a table, or an additional chair

Doing the Pose: Sitting close to the edge of the chair seat, extend your legs apart. Flex your ankles and firm your thighs. Place your hands in front of you on a wall, a table, or an additional chair. Keeping your sitting bones firmly rooted, with each inhalation press your hands to help lift taller through your spine and sternum. With each exhalation, fold slightly forward while trying to maintain the length of your spine. Breath by breath, explore folding farther forward. If after five to ten breaths it is comfortable in your low back and neck and you do not have advanced osteoporosis, explore allowing your spine to round. Hold for up to two minutes while breathing deeply.

Sunset Pose[1]

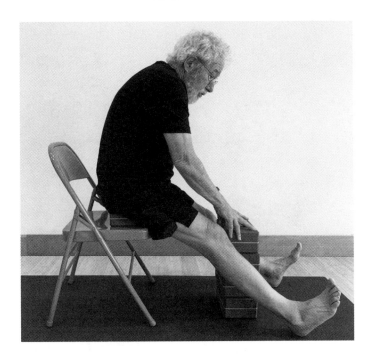

Special Sensitivity: Low back, neck. Contraindicated if you have advanced osteoporosis.

Props: Chair, possibly blocks and a blanket, and a wall, a table, or an additional chair

Doing the Pose: Sitting close to the edge of the chair seat, extend your legs straight forward. Flex your ankles and firm your thighs. Place your hands in front of you on a wall, a table, or an additional chair. Keeping your sitting bones firmly rooted, with each inhalation lift taller through your spine, using your hands to help create this upward movement (lifting your sternum away from your belly while drawing your pelvis down and back). With each exhalation, try to rotate your pelvis forward to draw your torso forward. Breath by breath, explore folding farther forward. If after five to ten breaths it is comfortable in your low back and neck and you do not have advanced osteoporosis, explore allowing your spine to round. Hold for up to two minutes while breathing deeply.

Inversion

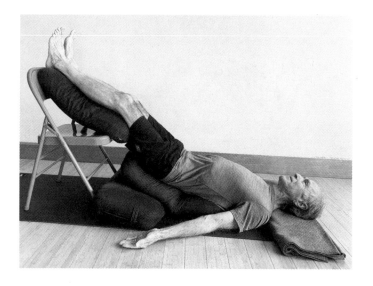

Special Sensitivity: Neck, low back

Props: Chair, possibly blocks, and a blanket or bolster

Doing the Pose: Coming to the floor, lie down on your back with a folded blanket or bolster placed under your pelvis (not low back) and your toes close to the front chair legs. Place one foot on the chair seat, then the other foot. Extend your legs up, placing your feet on the chair back. Relax your arms on the floor with your palms turned upward. Rest while breathing slowly for five to ten minutes.

Final Relaxation

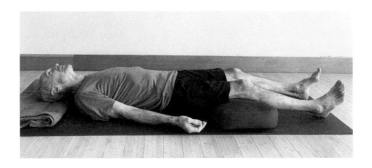

Special Sensitivity: Low back, neck

Props: Chair, possibly blocks, a blanket or bolster, and an eye pillow

Doing the Pose: Lie down on your back with your legs stretched out on the floor. Place a rolled blanket or bolster under your knees for greater overall comfort and ease in your low back. Relax through your legs, allowing your feet to comfortably turn out. With your arms draped on the floor by your sides, rest the backs of your hands on the floor, letting your shoulders relax down. Cover your eyes with an eye pillow (ideally aroma-free). Once you are entirely comfortable, take several deep breaths in and allow your breath to freely release out, feeling your body settling into the floor. Rest for five to ten minutes, allowing the breath to flow effortlessly and everything to let go.

Step 3: Chair Yoga Meditation Practices

See the meditation practices in chapters 4–6 (the practice in chapter 4 is for everyone, chapter 5 for anxiety or hyperarousal, and chapter 6 for depression or lethargy).

EPILOGUE

Daily and Nightly Rituals for Better Sleep

From ancient times to the present, in the East and West, much has been said, studied, and written about sleep. Priests and shamans, doctors and scientists, psychologists and New Age visionaries have offered their ideas about the nature of sleep, its purpose, and how to make it better. Over the ages, we have learned much yet also often forgotten much, especially as the refined insights of modern science have frequently overshadowed our personal and collective experience.

As with many other realms of contemporary life, with sleep we have tended to seek solutions in little pills that are easy to take yet carry potentially fateful consequences for our long-term well-being. The same pills that can help us to sleep can disturb the replenishing effects of sleep on the bodymind. Even the psychological strategies and tricks of cognitive behavioral therapy can take us further from the abiding truths of our lives that when illuminated can enable us to see more clearly how the ways we live our lives are very much at the heart of what ails us and what heals us.

Here we return the ancient wisdom of yogis and other seekers of truth and enlightenment whose understanding of light and dark, energy and lethargy, and sleep and wake states appreciates the natural pulsations of life. While in matters of sleep, our environment—our relationships, our work, our home, our planet—greatly matters and deserves attention, yoga points us more inside, to recognizing imbalances that cause difficulty. Health, joy, and love ultimately arise from within our own hearts, giving us the sustainable rhythms of life that make everything better, and make sleep happen more naturally and soundly.

This is the holistic view variously described across the ages with concepts such as kosha and *spanda,* the latter referring to the ceaseless vibrations of energy that permeate the universe and animate our being from deep in our own hearts. In following the kosha map of practice—nourishing our bodies, cultivating our life-force energies through the breath, opening and clearing our minds, letting our emotions open us to deeper wisdom, and living as the fully lovable and loving creatures we naturally are—we most easily relax, settle, and have better sleep.

In opening ourselves to discovering this loving energy at the core of our being—this spanda—everything in life changes. We accept ourselves as we are, even as we aim for greater self-cultivation. We accept others for who they are, even as we engage in sharing in ways that support mutual growth. We recognize that we are part of an amazing and ever-changing universe, including a universe of personal possibility, especially the possibility of thriving with full consciousness in this life.

The asana, pranayama, meditation, and visualization practices presented in this book are the essential yoga tools for bringing these qualities more to the fore in our daily lives. They give us ways to better understand and change the conditions of our lives that often disturb our sleep—conditions and sleep that science has gone far in helping us understand. For anyone with a complex life, confused thoughts, or unstable emotions, this self-understanding is part of a continuing daily project, with everything getting better one breath at a time.

With practice—ideally a daily routine—sleep and life are getting even better for all of us.

Waking in the morning, the sun close to the eastern horizon, you come into the renewed dawning of your wakeful consciousness. How do you feel? How did you sleep? If well, you are calm yet energized for meeting and greeting all that will come in the day. If your daily rhythms allow, you let the early light of day enter your eyes, strengthening your biological entrainment to the sun and your spiritual entrainment to the cosmos. A morning yoga practice is perfectly stimulating for you, for your conditions, allowing you to move into the fullness of the day with a greater sense of steadiness and ease. As your energy naturally drops in the early afternoon, you forgo the espresso or long nap in favor of a walk or a short asana-pranayama practice. If your yoga practice comes later in the day, it has a calming effect, delivering you into the evening with a sense of calm and contentment.

Now the sun is fading away, night is upon you, and you welcome the dark. Well before bedtime you create a sacred space for quieting your bodymind, perhaps lighting candles, sipping a calming tea, and reading your new favorite book. You are getting sleepy and it feels good. Your comfortable bed invites you in for a night of peaceful, restorative, nourishing sleep. Sweet dreams. *Namaste.*

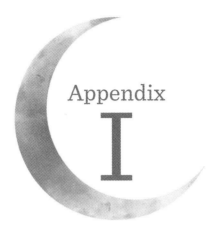

INTERNATIONAL CLASSIFICATION OF SLEEP DISORDERS[1]

Disorders marked with an asterisk coincide with the eleven sleep-wake disorders given in the *Diagnostic and Statistical Manual of Mental Disorders*, fifth edition (*DSM-V*).

Insomnia*

- Short-term insomnia
- Chronic insomnia
- Other insomnia (when insomnia symptoms do not meet criteria for the other two types of insomnia)

Sleep-Related Breathing Disorders

- Central sleep apnea syndromes*
  - Central sleep apnea with Cheyne–Stokes breathing
  - Central sleep apnea due to a medical disorder without Cheyne–Stokes breathing
  - Central sleep apnea due to high-altitude periodic breathing
  - Central sleep apnea due to a medication or substance
  - Primary central sleep apnea
  - Primary central sleep apnea of infancy
  - Primary central sleep apnea of prematurity
  - Treatment-emergent central sleep apnea
- Obstructive sleep apnea (OSA) syndromes*
  - OSA, adult
  - OSA, pediatric
- Sleep-related hypoventilation disorders*
  - Obesity hypoventilation syndrome
  - Congenital central alveolar hypoventilation syndrome
  - Late-onset central hypoventilation with hypothalamic dysfunction
  - Idiopathic central alveolar hypoventilation
  - Sleep-related hypoventilation due to a medication or substance
  - Sleep-related hypoventilation due to a medical disorder
  - Sleep-related hypoxemia disorder

- Isolated symptoms and normal variants
  - Snoring
  - Catathrenia

Central Disorders of Hypersomnolence*

- Narcolepsy type 1*
- Narcolepsy type 2*
- Idiopathic hypersomnia
- Kleine–Levin syndrome
- Hypersomnia due to a medical disorder
- Hypersomnia due to a medication or substance
- Hypersomnia associated with a psychiatric disorder
- Insufficient sleep syndrome

Circadian Rhythm Sleep-Wake Disorders*

- Delayed sleep-wake phase disorder
- Advanced sleep-wake phase disorder
- Irregular sleep-wake rhythm disorder
- Non-24-hour sleep-wake rhythm disorder
- Shift work disorder
- Jet lag disorder
- Circadian sleep-wake disorder not otherwise specified

Parasomnias

- NREM-related parasomnias
  - Disorder of arousal from NREM sleep*
  - Confusional arousals
  - Sleepwalking
  - Sleep terrors
  - Sleep-related eating disorder
- REM-related parasomnias
  - REM sleep behavior disorder*
  - Recurrent isolated sleep paralysis
  - Nightmare disorder*
- Other parasomnias
  - Exploding head syndrome
  - Sleep-related hallucinations
  - Sleep enuresis
  - Parasomnia due to a medical disorder
  - Parasomnia due to a medication or substance
  - Parasomnia, unspecified

Sleep-Related Movement Disorders

- Restless legs syndrome*
- Periodic limb movement disorder
- Sleep-related leg cramps
- Sleep-related bruxism

- Sleep-related rhythmic movement disorder
- Benign sleep myoclonus of infancy
- Propriospinal myoclonus at sleep onset
- Sleep-related movement disorder due to a medical disorder
- Sleep-related movement disorder due to a medication or substance*
- Sleep-related movement disorder, unspecified

Other Sleep Disorders

- Isolated symptoms and normal variants—other sleep-related symptoms or events that do not meet the standard definition of a sleep disorder
- Some occur during normal sleep. As an example, sleep talking occurs at some time in most normal sleepers.
- Some lie on the continuum between normal and abnormal. As an example, snoring without associated airway compromise, sleep disturbance, or other consequences is essentially normal, whereas heavy snoring is often part of obstructive sleep apnea.

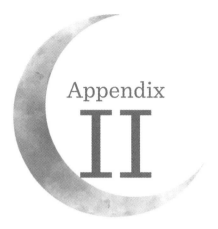

Appendix

II

SLEEP ASSESSMENT

Yoga Self-Assessment

For detailed guidance in doing self-assessment related to general physical conditions and in relation to asana, pranayama, and meditation practices, see my book *Yoga Therapy*.[1] The same guidelines are here: *www.markstephensyoga.com/yogaforbettersleep.selfassessment*.

In doing yoga self-assessment, start by reflecting on where you are in your daily life with respect to the yamas and niyamas discussed in chapter 3. Write each of the five yamas and five niyamas at the top of separate pages in a personal journal. Write whatever comes to you, giving greater attention to those that might feel troubling. Do one at a time.

After a few minutes of this self-reflective journaling, put your journal aside and come to a comfortable upright sitting position with your eyes resting lightly closed. Tune into the breath, visualizing the inhalations flowing directly into your heart center, and visualizing the exhalations fading out behind you like the wake of a boat. Begin breathing your journal reflections into your heart, into the infinitely spacious love in your heart. With each exhalation, allow what you are feeling to fade out behind you. Keep doing this with just that one feeling, with each breath getting more deeply into it, its source, its effects in your life, its reality, and keep letting it go. As you stay with it, imagine any negative power of the feeling softening in your heart, attenuating, letting go.

Now come back to your journal and add whatever seems important or insightful to your page. Then go to each of the next yamas, then each niyama. Breath by breath, tuning in and letting go, allow this to deepen your svadyaya.

Sleep Diary

Use these questions to discover more about your sleep patterns and experiences. Use the Sleep Log to track some of these patterns and experiences over a period of a few weeks.

1. What time did you wish to wake up this morning? What time did you wake up?

2. What caused you to awaken in the morning?

3. Did you awaken during the night? If so, was it due to needing to urinate?

4. What did you do during the last two hours before you went to bed?

5. How did you feel during the day (mood, drowsiness, etc.)? Why?

6. What time did you begin and end any daytime naps?

7. What medications did you take during the day (sleeping pills, caffeine, and alcohol)?

8. When did you eat dinner, and what did you eat?

9. What did you do in the last hour before going to bed?

10. How stressed (if at all) were you before going to bed, and why?

11. When did you go to bed?

12. When do you think you fell asleep?

13. What can you recall thinking or doing in the last few minutes before falling asleep?

14. If you woke during the night, why? How many times? How long did it take to fall back asleep?

15. How well do you feel you slept? How rested do you feel?

16. How were your dreams?

Sleep Log

	MON.	TUES.	WED.	THURS.	FRI.	SAT.	SUN.
Complete When You Awake in the Morning:							
Time you went to bed							
Time you got out of bed							
Hours slept							
Number of times you awoke during the night							
Complete Before Going to Bed:							
Did you do yoga today?							
Minutes you exercised today							

	MON.	TUES.	WED.	THURS.	FRI.	SAT.	SUN.
Activity during the two hours before going to bed							
Number of caffeinated drinks today							
Number of alcoholic drinks within three hours of going to bed							
How was your energy today? (1–10)							
How was your mood today? (1–10)							

Conventional Sleep Assessment Tools

If you wish to go further in your sleep assessments, consider using one or several of the different assessment instruments taken from sleep medicine and sleep psychology sources. Each tool can be found by referring to the endnote.

- The Insomnia Severity Index assesses sleep quality, fatigue, psychological symptoms, and quality of life.[2]

- The Pittsburgh Sleep Quality Index provides a questionnaire to evaluate clinically derived sleep difficulties related to quality, latency, duration, habitual efficiency, sleep disturbances, use of sleep medication, and daytime dysfunction.[3]

- The Multidimensional Fatigue Inventory measures general fatigue, mental fatigue, physical fatigue, reduced activity, and reduced motivation using a five-point Likert scale.[4]

- The Beck Depression Inventory consists of a twenty-one-item questionnaire measuring depressive and anxiety symptoms in the past week (both anxiety and depression are measured due to their frequent co-occurrence).[5]

- The Beck Anxiety Inventory consists of a twenty-one-item questionnaire measuring anxiety symptoms in the past week.[6]

- The State-Trait Anxiety Inventory assesses situational (state) versus general (trait) qualities of anxiety.[7]

- The SF-12 Health Survey questionnaire has twelve items in eight health domains: physical functioning, role physical (limitation in routine activities due to physical conditions), bodily pain, general health, vitality, social functioning, role emotional (limitation in routine activities due to emotional conditions), and mental health.[8]

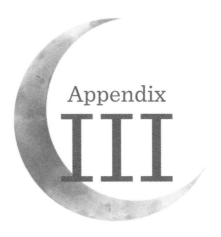

TIPS FOR BETTER SLEEP[1]

1. **Stick to a sleep schedule.** Go to bed and wake up at the same time each day. As creatures of habit, people have a hard time adjusting to changes in sleep patterns. Sleeping later on weekends won't fully make up for a lack of sleep during the week and will make it harder to wake up early on Monday morning.

2. **Exercise is great, but not too late in the day.** Try to exercise at least thirty minutes on most days but not later than two to three hours before your bedtime.

3. **Avoid caffeine and nicotine before bed.** Coffee, colas, certain teas, and chocolate contain the stimulant caffeine, and its effects can take as long as eight hours to wear off fully. Therefore, a cup of coffee in the late afternoon can

make it hard for you to fall asleep at night. Nicotine is also a stimulant, often causing smokers to sleep only very lightly. In addition, smokers often wake up too early in the morning because of nicotine withdrawal.

4. **Avoid alcoholic drinks before bed.** Having a "nightcap" or alcoholic beverage before sleep may help you relax, but heavy use robs you of deep sleep and REM sleep, keeping you in the lighter stages of sleep. Heavy alcohol ingestion also may contribute to breathing impairment at night. You also tend to wake up in the middle of the night when the effects of the alcohol have worn off.

5. **Avoid large meals and beverages late at night.** A light snack is okay, but a large meal can cause indigestion that interferes with sleep. Drinking too many fluids at night can cause frequent awakenings to urinate.

6. **If possible, avoid medicines that delay or disrupt your sleep.** Some commonly prescribed heart, blood pressure, or asthma medications, as well as some over-the-counter and herbal remedies for coughs, colds, or allergies, can disrupt sleep patterns. If you have trouble sleeping, talk to your healthcare provider or pharmacist to see whether any drugs you're taking might be contributing to your insomnia and ask whether they can be taken at other times during the day or early in the evening.

7. **Don't take naps after 3 p.m.** Naps can help make up for lost sleep, but late afternoon naps can make it harder to fall asleep at night.

8. **Relax before bed.** Don't overschedule your day so that no time is left for unwinding. A relaxing activity, such as reading or listening to music, should be part of your bedtime ritual.

9. **Take a hot bath before bed.** The drop in body temperature after getting out of the bath may help you feel sleepy, and the bath can help you relax and slow down so you're more ready to sleep.

10. **Have a good sleeping environment.** Get rid of anything in your bedroom that might distract you from sleep, such as noises, bright lights, an uncomfortable bed, or warm temperatures. You sleep better if the temperature in the room is kept cool. A TV, cell phone, or computer in the bedroom can be a distraction and deprive you of needed sleep. Having a comfortable mattress and pillow can help promote a good night's sleep. Individuals who have insomnia often watch the clock. Turn the clock's face out of view so you don't worry about the time while trying to fall asleep.

11. **Have the right sunlight exposure.** Daylight is key to regulating daily sleep patterns. Try to get outside in natural sunlight for at least thirty minutes each day. If possible, wake up with the sun or use bright room lights in the morning. Sleep experts recommend that, if you have problems falling asleep, you should get an hour of exposure to morning sunlight and turn down the lights before bedtime.

12. **Don't lie in bed awake.** If you find yourself still awake after staying in bed for more than 30 minutes or if you are starting to feel anxious or worried, get up and do some relaxing activity until you feel sleepy. The anxiety of not being able to sleep can make it harder to fall asleep.

13. **See a health professional if you continue to have trouble sleeping.** If you consistently find it difficult to fall or stay asleep and/or feel tired or not well rested during

the day despite spending enough time in bed at night, you may have a sleep disorder. Your family healthcare provider or a sleep specialist should be able to help you, and it is important to rule out other health or emotional problems that may be disturbing your sleep.

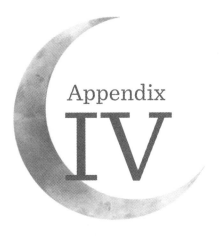

TIPS FOR JET LAG AND SHIFT WORK

Jet lag, including the "social jet lag" that happens to most of us on nonworking weekends and holidays, and shift work misalign our bodies and the day/night cycles at our place on the planet, making us sleepy when we need to be awake and awake when our body wishes to be sleeping. These strategies for better sleeping and waking can be effective in getting better sleep.

Jet Lag

- In the week prior to traveling, try to gradually adjust your time in bed toward the sleep-wake times of your destination.

- If flying east to west for more than six hours, try to take a night flight and allow yourself to go to sleep as soon as possible on the flight. Try using noise-canceling headphones with soothing music, and wear a blindfold. After six hours, wake up, get light exposure (try to have a window seat), and try to stay awake until close to bedtime at your destination.

- Limit naps to less than two hours.

- Do not consume caffeine within three hours of bedtime.

- As an alternative to a night flight, try to take a flight that arrives in the early evening, then stay up until 10 or 11 p.m.

- Upon arrival (or while still en route), try to expose yourself to light on the schedule of your destination time zone. If on an airplane, consider using an LED screen for light exposure.

- Once at your destination, try to get out of bed and into natural sunlight in the morning and during as much of the day as you can. Eat on the schedule of your new location.

- Exercise to stimulate circulation and promote energy. Try to do a stimulating morning yoga practice (try the sequences given in chapter 6).

- Relax when you are wound up. Try the sequences given in chapter 5 if it is close to bedtime and you are not tired.

- Consider using melatonin for the first few nights only. Minimize alcohol consumption, and definitely do not use alcohol as a sleep sedative.

- Sleep. Even if sleeping causes you to more slowly adjust to your new time zone, healthy sleep ultimately allows a healthier overall adjustment to your new environment.

Shift Work

- Try to maintain consistent sleep-wake times, including on days off.

- Try to avoid frequently rotating shifts. If you have a temporarily rotated shift, use bright light in your workplace to help stay alert.

- If you have a rotating shift, if possible try to have your shifts rotate clockwise, in the direction of day shift to evening shift to night shift.

- If you know of an upcoming change in your shift schedule, try to gradually shift your sleep-wake schedule in that direction three days prior to the change occurring.

- Minimize consumption of caffeine. If you must consume caffeine (or other stimulants), try to consume it early in your wake phase and as far from bedtime as tolerable.

- Add blackout curtains to your sleep paradise and give clear instruction to not be disturbed.

- Do the yoga sequence given in chapter 4 before going to bed. Do the yoga sequence in chapter 6 soon after waking.

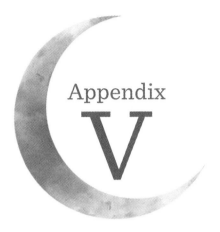

Appendix

V

ADDITIONAL SLEEP RESOURCES

Mark Stephens Yoga: *www.MarkStephensYoga.com*

> Find extensive information on doing yoga postures, breathing exercises, and meditation: spoken word, video, articles, quotes, poetry, and more. The primary focus of the website is on teaching yoga, including basic and advanced teacher training and continuing education for new and experienced yoga teachers.

North Atlantic Books: *www.northatlanticbooks.com*

> An independent, nonprofit publisher committed to a bold exploration of the relationships between body, mind, spirit, and nature. Find a diverse range of original books in alternative medicine, ecology, and spirituality, with a pioneering publishing program that encompasses somatics, trauma, raw foods, craniosacral therapy, shamanism, and literature.

National Sleep Foundation: *www.sleepfoundation.org*

> As a global voice for sleep health, the National Sleep Foundation is dedicated to improving health and well-being through education and advocacy.

Stanford University Division of Sleep Medicine: *www.med .stanford.edu/sleepdivision.html*

> Since starting the world's first sleep clinic and laboratory in 1972, Stanford Sleep Medicine Center has emerged as the foremost international center for the study of sleep and the management of sleep disorders.

Harvard University Division of Sleep Medicine: *www.healthysleep .med.harvard.edu*

> Find the latest information on why sleep matters, the science of sleep, and strategies for getting the sleep you need.

GLOSSARY OF KEY TERMS

abhyasa: Perseverance in one's self-cultivation, in doing yoga. It is one side of the coin. For the other side, see vairagya.

adenosine: The primary neuromodulator that promotes sleep and suppresses arousal. Caffeine binds to its receptors in the brain, blocking it from functioning.

ahimsa: To be in life without hurting oneself or others; nonviolence. The first yama.

alpha waves: The slow brain wave pattern when conscious and relaxed.

antara kumbhaka: The natural pause or suspension of movement in the breath when filled with breath. Also refers to holding the breath in once the lungs are full.

aparigraha: To be open to life's experiences without grasping for things that are not naturally coming to you or arising within you; noncovetousness. The fifth yama.

apnea: The involuntary cessation of breathing when filled with breath.

asana: Posture. More specifically, to be steady, at ease, and present when in a posture and when transitioning in and out of it.

asteya: Not stealing; not taking what is not yours. The third yama.

avidyā: Ignorance, especially of the true nature of things and thoughts.

bahya kumbhaka: The natural pause or suspension of movement in the breath when empty of breath. Also refers to holding the breath out once the lungs are empty.

bhastrika: Literally, "bellows"; a breathing technique in which the breath is quickly and forcefully moved through the nostrils without interruption.

beta waves: The brain waves when alert and in normal waking consciousness.

brahmacharya: In ancient yoga writings, this means sexual celibacy. In modern yoga parlance, it refers to "right use of energy," particularly one's own sexual energy. The fifth yama. It is best considered in relation to the other yamas.

chitta vrtti nirodha: To still the fluctuations of the mind.

circadian rhythm: When biological processes—such as the release of melatonin—oscillate generally in entrainment to the twenty-four-hour clock and with greater refinement from environmental cues such as light and temperature (called zeitgebers, "time givers").

delta waves: High-amplitude brain waves associated with deep sleep.

dharana: A focused meditative state. Also, the practice for attaining dhyana. A niyama.

dhyana: A purely contemplative state, beyond a concentrated mind. A niyama.

homeostasis: Maintenance of relative stability in the interrelated physiological process of an organism, including the human organism.

hyperarousal: A state of heightened stress and anxiety often associated with post-traumatic stress disorder (PTSD).

ishvara-pranidhana: Opening to and reflecting upon one's life as part of the larger forces of the universe. The fifth niyama.

kleshas: Mental and emotional afflictions that disturb the mind.

melatonin: A hormone secreted by the pineal gland that is triggered by darkness. Rising levels of melatonin are a major factor associated with sleep onset and sleep maintenance.

nadi: Energy channel through which prana flows.

nadi shodhana: Alternate nostril breathing. Generally calming, especially with lengthened exhalations.

niyama: Ancient precepts for cultivating a pure quality of being. See saucha, samtosa, tapas, svadyaya, and ishvara-pranidhana.

NREM: Non-rapid eye movement. There is little to no dreaming during NREM sleep. There are four stages of NREM sleep, N1–N4, with N3/N4 being the deepest (as measured by difficulty in being aroused).

pada bandha: The energetic action of rooting down through the legs and feet to activate intrinsic foot and lower leg muscles that support the arches and ankles.

parasympathetic nervous system: The part of the autonomic nervous system associated with relaxation. Sometimes called the rest and digest system. It promotes sleep.

pineal gland: A small, pinecone-shaped, melatonin-producing endocrine gland located in a groove near the center of the brain. It receives light-stimulated signals from the suprachiasmatic nucleus that relate sleep-inducing melatonin to the light/dark cycles of the day and night.

playing the edge: A technique in yoga in which one uses breath phases with internal sensations (interoception and proprioception) to consciously explore tension and relaxation in actively opening to deeper yet more stable and relaxed experiences of asanas and pranayamas.

prana: Life-force energy.

pranayama: Various conscious breathing techniques that have different effects on internal energy, awareness, and mood.

pratyahara: To relieve oneself of external sensory stimuli. Also described as the willful suspension of the cognitive apparatus.

Process C: Circadian regulation of the body's internal processes that partially drives the tendencies to sleep and wake. It functions in relation to independent Process S in sleep-wake regulation.

Process S: Homeostatic sleep drive generated by the accumulation of sleep-inducing substances in the brain.

REM: Rapid eye movement. One of five sleep phases. In REM sleep, also known as paradoxical sleep, is distinguished by rapid movement of the eyes beneath the eyelids, muscle atonia, and dreams. Not to be confused with a pioneering alternative rock band from Athens, Georgia, whose debut single, "Radio Free Europe," was released in 1981 to critical acclaim.

saucha: Purity. An active practice of cultivating purity of body-mind. The first of the five niyamas.

sleep pressure: The accumulation of sleep-inducing factors to make us sleepy. See Process C and Process S.

samadhi: A state of pure consciousness unaffected by conditions of the bodymind. The eighth limb of the eight-limb yoga path (ashtanga yoga). It is attained by virtue of practicing the seven prior limbs with abhyasa and vairagya.

samtosa: Contentment. The second niyama.

satya: Truth. The second yama.

sleep maintenance insomnia: Difficulty staying asleep.

sleep onset insomnia: Difficulty falling asleep.

sleep pressure: The accumulation of homeostatic forces that make us sleepy. See adenosine.

sthira sukham asanam: Steadiness, ease, and presence of mind. The definition of asana given in Patañjali's Yoga Sūtra.

suprachiasmatic nucleus: A set of tiny light-sensitive nuclei located above the optic chiasm in the hypothalamus of the brain. It receives light data from the optic nerve and relays it to the pineal gland, entraining the production and release of melatonin to light.

svadyaya: Self-study. The fourth niyama.

sympathetic nervous system: The part of the autonomic nervous system associated with automatically reactive physiological changes and behaviors. Activates what is sometimes called the fight-or-flight response. Associated with difficulty in sleep onset and maintenance.

tapas: Austere and self-disciplined action in doing yoga. The third niyama. Not to be confused with traditional Spanish food.

theta waves: Electrical activity in the hippocampus of the brain thought by some to be associated with clear awareness as when in a pure meditative state. The associations and effects of theta waves vary in different animals. The ethics of human-subject research in relation to the location of theta waves in the hippocampus have limited their assessment. There is some evidence that theta waves are associated with NREM stage N1, what ancient yoga literature calls yoga nidra.

ujjayi: Uplifting or victorious. Ujjayi pranayama is the basic technique of breathing in yoga.

vairagya: By way of nonattachment. For the other side of the yoga practice coin, see abhyasa.

viloma: Literally, "anti-hair." A pranayama technique. Refers to going against the natural tendency of the breath flow in and out by holding the breath one to five times during both inhalation and exhalation.

vrtti: Fluctuate. Refers to the fluctuation of the mind (thinking) or the breath (as in sama and visama vrtti pranayama techniques). See chitta vrtti nirodha.

yama: To contain. The first limb of ashtanga yoga, referring to cultivation of one's moral container.

NOTES

Preface

1 Stranges et al. (2012, 1173–81), Blanco et al. (2004, 155–59).

2 U.S. Centers for Disease Control and Prevention (2014), Leger et al. (2008, 307–17).

3 To be clear, most people today do not think they must bow to the east or otherwise pay homage to a sun god to ensure the sun's "return" at dawn, as astrophysics has done a pretty good job explaining such cosmic phenomena. Nor are we inclined to moderate our impulses by wrecking our tissues through self-mortification (alcohol, drug, and nicotine abuse aside). We also understand that the concept found in yoga and especially Ayurveda of ether as a fundamental component of the universe is archaic and mythical, not something with which to explain the nature of the universe, human beings, or health.

Chapter 1

1 To explore the world of goddesses in yoga and tantra, with stories we can invoke on our personal paths of transformation, see Kempton (2013, 2014).

2 Wilkins (2003, 48–52).

3 Roebuck (2003, 347–48), Sharma (2004).

4 The insights of ancient yoga philosophy, theory, and practice arise from direct experience, intuition, speculation, and claims of divine transmission, sources and methods that generally do not meet the standards of inquiry and evidence assumed in modern nonreligious understanding. Thus, we find many postulates and practices that are

unclear, contradictory, and lacking efficacy. We should not blame the ancient seers and writers for such theoretical, methodological, and empirical limitation (while holding contemporary sources accountable for their ideas), nor should we accept their misunderstandings and ill-informed practices because of their limitations.

5 Steriade and McCarley (2005, 188). On the neural processes controlling sleep and wake states, see Brown et al. (2012).

6 Buzsáki and Draguhn (2004, 1926–29).

7 Kahana (2006, 1669–72).

8 Jones (2003, 438–51).

9 Raichle et al. (2001, 676–82). On pratyahara and dharana, see early Buddhist and yogic views, respectively, in Gyatso (2004) and Woods (2003).

10 Jacobs and Azmitia (1992, 165–229), Jones (1993, 61–71), Lin (2000, 471–503).

11 Borbély (1982, 195–204), Borbély et al. (2016, 131–43).

12 Basheer et al. (2004, 379–96), Dunwiddie and Masino (2001, 31–55).

13 Gautier-Sauvigné et al. (2005, 101–13).

14 Hayaishi et al. (2004, 533–39), Huang et al. (2007, 33–38), Imeri and Opp (2009, 199–210).

15 Borbély and Achermann (1999, 557–68).

16 Saper, Scammell, and Lu (2005, 1257–63).

17 Descartes (1993), Lokhorst (2017).

18 Blavatsky (1933, 293–94). The Theosophists are not alone in distorting the pineal gland and many other things in the yoga realm, as we can see in the imaginative pseudoscience found in contemporary writings about yoga and the pineal gland. For self-edification or entertainment, read the results of an internet search using the search terms "yoga pineal gland," and you will find just about anything you wish to imagine or believe.

19 Roenneberg et al. (2003, 80–90).

20 Lucas et al. (2012, 1–18), Moore (1983, 2783–89). Melatonin also helps regulate blood pressure and may play an antioxidant role in the immune system. See Roenneberg (2007, 429–38).

21 Aserinsky and Kleitman (1953, 273–74), Dement and Kleitman (1957b, 339–46).

22 Jones (2005, 136–53).

23 Rechtschaffen and Kales (1968).

24 For the *Mandukya Upanishad,* see Roebuck (2003, 347–48). See chapter 3 for yoga nidra meditation practices to help with sleep. See also Satyananda Saraswati (1976).

25 Amzica (1992, 285–94).

26 Domhoff (2018).

27 Aserinsky and Kleitman (1953, 273–74), Dement and Kleitman (1957a, 673–90).

28 There are different and often contending views of the science, most significantly in the cognitive versus activation-synthesis debate. See Foulkes and Domhoff (2014, 168–71), Domhoff (2018), and Walker (2017, 199–206).

29 Luppi et al. (2013, 1–7).

30 There is increasing evidence that memory consolidation occurs more in NREM and REM, contrary to the dominant view of Allan Hobson, Alice Stickland, and others. See Payne (2010, 101–34).

31 McCarley et al. (1983, 359–64), Wehrle et al. (2007, 863–71).

32 Jouvet (1962, 125–206).

33 Schenck et al. (1986, 293–308).

34 Muscle tension almost completely subsides when we are sleeping, due to muscle atonia, such that there are few if any motor neurons firing when we sleep. Without motor neurons firing into skeletal muscle tissues, there cannot be muscular tension in them. These facts have not kept some leading yoga voices from asserting that tense muscles do not relax when sleeping, claiming it causes us to wake with a headache or clenched jaw, but this is incorrect (except in certain pathological conditions).

35 Hirshkowitz and Schmidt (2005, 311–29), Abel et al. (1979, 5–14), Rogers et al. (1985, 327–42).

36 It is beyond the scope of this book to explicate REM control mechanisms, which include cholinergic and aminergic mechanisms (key elements in the reciprocal interaction model), GABAergic control, and nitric oxide control. To explore, see McCarley (2004, 429–67), Hobson et al. (1975, 55–58).

37 Saper, Cano, and Scammell (2005, 92–98).

38 Freud (1994 [1899]), Jung (2002), Perls (1973).

39 Foulkes and Domhoff (2014), Domhoff (2018), Walker and Stickgold (2006, 139–66).

40 For example, Walker (2009, 168–97).

41 Some claim the ancient texts are from seers who gained insight through a supernatural medium, from God or the gods, which could be, this despite an abundance of fundamental errors in explaining physical reality, from the nature of the body to the nature of the cosmos.

42 What follows is drawn from Roebuck (2003, 464–65).

43 Sharma (2004). On the rise of the *Yoga Sūtra* to prominence after centuries of obscurity or irrelevance, see White (2012b).

44 Satyananda Saraswati (1976).

45 Walker (2017, 108).

46 Less than six hours of sleep is not unhealthy only for a tiny percentage of people who possess the rare BHLHE41/DEC2 gene. Then there are the rest of us, who are fooling ourselves if we think we are okay with a little amount, or think that we can catch up on the weekends. Walker (2017, 261), Kurien et al. (2013, 873–79), Fulda and Schulz (2001, 423–45).

47 Ellenbogen (2005, E25–E27), Walker (2008, S29–S34), Killgore (2010, 105–29).

48 Muzur et al. (2002, 475–81).

49 Mander et al. (2011, 183–84), Mander et al. (2015, 1051–57), Kaida et al. (2015, 72–79), Payne (2010, 101–34).

50 Born and Wilhelm (2012, 192–203), Diekelmann and Born (2010, 114–26), Buzsáki (1989, 551–70).

51 Goldstein-Piekarski et al. (2015, 10135–45), van der Helm et al. (2010, 335–42).

52 Astill et al. (2014, 910), Kuriyama et al. (2004, 705–13).

53 Walker et al. (2002, 205–11).

54 Vinters (2015, 291–319).

55 Storandt et al. (2006, 467–73).

56 Walker (2017, 160).

57 Nedergaard and Goldman (2016, 44–49), Plog and Nedergaard (2018, 379–94).

Chapter 2

1 Buysse (2014, 9–17).

2 American Academy of Sleep Medicine (2014), American Psychiatric Association (2013).

3 Ohayon and Reynolds (2009, 952–60). See especially tables 3, 4, and 5.

4 The 30–35 percent figure is found in numerous studies of the adult population, including in societies as different as India and the United States, while others find slightly higher percentages, often with somewhat different measures of what constitutes insomnia. For example, Morin et al. (2006, 123–30), Bhaskar et al. (2016, 780–84), Walker (2017, 240–41).

5 The yoga prism through which we look here is primarily the yoga philosophy and psychology presented in the *Yoga Sūtra of Patañjali,* from around 325 BCE. On the science, for a general introduction, see Schwartz and Kilduff (2015, 615–44), Brown and McKenna (2015, 135).

6 Neckelmann et al. (2007, 873–80), Harvey (2001, 1037–59).

7 Germain (2013, 372–82), Babson and Feldner (2010, 1–15), Singareddy and Balon (2002, 183–90).

8 Elklit et al. (2014), Hall Brown and Mellman (2014, 198–206), Belleville et al. (2011, 318–27), Van der Kolk (1984, 187–90).

9 Bonnet and Arand (2010, 9–15).

10 American Psychiatric Association (2013).

11 Wiegand et al. (2002, 251).

12 Kurlansik and Ibay (2012, 1037–41), LoBello and Mehta (2018, 72–79).

13 Harvey et al. (2015, 564–77).

14 Finan et al. (2013, 1539–52).

15 Smith and Haythornthwaite (2004, 119–32).

16 Tang (2008, 2–7).

17 It is worth noting that most of the top mass-circulation books on sleep written by neuroscientists, sleep medicine scientists, and research and clinical psychologists fail to address physical pain as a significant factor in insomnia, or never address it at all, this despite 40 percent of people with insomnia having chronic physical pain. See Glovinsky and Spielman (2006 and 2017), Jacobs (1998), Walker (2017), and Winter (2017).

18 Brooks and Canal (2013, 551–60).

19 Bes et al. (1991, 5–12).

20 Kurth et al. (2010, 13211–19), Taylor et al. (2005, 239–44).

21 Carskadon (2011, 637–47).

22 Hansen et al. (2005, 1555–61).

23 Monk (2005, 366–74).

24 Walker (2017, 97–98).

25 Neikrug and Ancoli-Israel (2010, 181–89), Duffy et al. (1998, R1478–R1487).

26 Mander et al. (2017, 19–36).

27 Freedman and Roehrs (2007, 826–29), Young et al. (2003, 667–72).

28 Lack et al. (2009, 1–8).

29 Fowler et al. (2017, 2548–61), Thornton et al. (2017, 1–9).

30 Beers (2000, 33–40).

31 Czeisler (1995, 254–302), Khalsa et al. (2003, 945–52).

32 Akerstedt et al. (2002, 585–88), Budnick et al. (1994, 1295–300), Richardson et al. (1989, 265–73), Pilcher and Coplen (2000, 573–88).

33 Knutsson (2003, 103–8), Folkard (1989, 182–86).

34 Yumino et al. (2009, 279–85).

35 White (2012a, 1363–70).

36 Katz et al. (1990, 1228–31).

37 This annual figure is steadily dropping since a high of more than 255 million in 2012. U.S. Centers for Disease Control and Prevention (2019).

38 Hasler et al. (2004, 661–66).

39 Shamsuzzaman et al. (2003, 1906–14).

40 Macey et al. (2008, 967–77).

41 Ohayon and Roth (2002, 547–54).

42 Ekbom and Ulfberg (2009, 419–31).

43 Plante and Winkelman (2006, 969–87).

44 Stores (2007, 405–17), Schenck et al. (1986, 293–308).

45 Ohayon et al. (1999, 268–76), Pressman (2007, 5–30).

46 Seeman (2011, 59–67).

47 Kales et al. (1980, 1413–17).

48 Gehrman and Harb (2010, 1185–94).

49 Andersen et al. (2007, 271–82), Dubessy et al. (2017).

50 Pearce (1989, 907–10).

51 Siclari et al. (2010, 3494–95).

52 Sharpless and Barber (2011, 311–15).

53 Scammell (2003, 154–66).

54 Boutrel and Koob (2004, 1183–90), Frary et al. (2005, 110–13).

55 Stein and Friedmann (2005, 1–13).

56 Daly and Fredholm (1998, 199–206), Benowitz (1990, 277–88).

57 Haskell et al. (2005, 813–25).

58 Bchir et al. (2006, 512–19), Drake et al. (2013, 1195–200).

59 Mosqueda-Garcia et al. (1993, 157–76), Nardi et al. (2009, 149–53).

60 Singh et al. (2009, 115–26).

61 Boutrel and Koob (2004, 1189–94).

62 Given that more than two-thirds of the *DSM-V* Task Force were psychiatrists with direct ties to the pharmaceutical industry, it is worth pondering how these ties and the specialized medical background of psychiatrists might be related to the preponderance of prescription medication treatments in addressing nearly every sleep disorder, among both children and adults.

63 Roebuck (2003, 357), Monier-Williams (1899, 438).

64 Monier-Williams (1899, 1135).

65 Dew et al. (2003, 63–73).

66 Heslop et al. (2002, 305–14), Kronholm et al. (2011, 215–21).

67 Ford and Kamerow (1989, 1479–84).

68 Krause et al. (2017, 404–18), Gujar et al. (2010, 1637–48).

69 Cole (2009, 3418–19), Chennaoui et al. (2011, 318–24), Conlon et al. (2007, 182–83), Haus and Smolensky (2013, 273–84).

70 Cappuccio et al. (2011, 1484–92), Fernandez-Mendoza et al. (2012, 929–35), Hall et al. (2004, 56–62).

71 Stranges et al. (2010, 896–902), Ayas et al. (2003, 205–9).

72 Slavich and Irwin (2014, 774–815), Gangwisch et al. (2010, 62–69).

73 Gangwisch et al. (2005, 1289–96), Kubo et al. (2011, 327–31), Cappuccio et al. (2008, 619–26), Buxton and Marcelli (2010, 1027–36).

74 Engeda et al. (2013, 676–80), Kawakami et al. (2004, 282–83).

75 Dinges et al. (1997, 267–77), Bernert and Joiner (2007, 735–43), Kamphuis et al. (2012, 327–34).

76 Besedovsky et al. (2012, 121–37), Lange et al. (2010, 48–59), Cohen et al. (2009, 62–67).

77 Astill et al. (2014, 910), Folkard and Åkersted (2004, A161–A167), Barger et al. (2005, 15–34).

Chapter 3

1 McKenna (2007, 245–52), Venkatraman et al. (2007, 603–9).

2 Buysse (2014, 9–17).

3 If you have chronic insomnia, a sleep-related breathing disorder, or another health problem that might be the cause of sleep disturbance, it might behoove you to obtain professional assessment. Sleep medicine labs are equipped with polysomnography tools to measure sleep onset, continuity, and architecture (NREM stages and REM), while actigraphy tools are utilized to assess sleep in one's natural sleep setting.

4 Buysse (2014, 12–13).

5 Walker (2017, 271–75).

6 Roehrs and Roth (2001, 101–9).

7 Ebrahim et al. (2013, 539–49).

8 Gaoni and Mechoulam (1964, 1646–47), Mechoulam et al. (2002, 11S–19S), Mechoulam and Parker (2013, 1363–64).

9 Backes (2014, 42–52).

10 Abrams and Guzman (2008, 246–84).

11 Backes (2014, 42–45).

12 On the effects of CBD, see Mechoulam et al. (2002, 11S–19S), Blessing et al. (2015, 825–36), Mead (2017, 288–91). As of January 1, 2019, hemp containing not more than 0.3 percent THC is legal in the United States. See U.S. Congress (2019).

13 Chong et al. (2013).

14 Aaron Beck, building on the work of Alfred Adler and others, is credited with pioneering cognitive behavioral therapy. See Beck (1975).

15 Wilson (2010, 1577–1601).

16 Okajima et al. (2011, 24–34), Bélanger et al. (2016, 659–67).

17 Fancher (1995).

18 Harvey (2000, 53–55).

19 Wilson (2017).

20 Olff et al. (2013, 1883–94), Sobrinho (2003, 35–39).

21 Zeitzer et al. (2000, 695–702).

22 Lack et al. (2008, 307–17), Gubin et al. (2017, 632–49).

23 Muzet (2007, 135–42), Griefahn et al. (2008, 569–77), Amundsen et al. (2013, 3921–28).

24 Gangwisch (2009, 37–45), Arble et al. (2010, 785–800).

25 Spiegel et al. (2009, 253–61).

26 St.-Onge et al. (2016, 19–24).

27 Cappuccio et al. (2008, 619–26).

28 Cota et al. (2006, 85–107).

29 Youngstedt (2005, 355–65).

30 Montgomery et al. (1985, 69–74), Driver et al. (1994, 903–7).

31 Myllymaki et al. (2011, 146–53), Shapiro et al. (1985, 624–27).

32 Flausino et al. (2012, 186–92).

33 Stephens (2017), Khalsa et al. (2016), Balasubramaniam et al. (2013, 1–16), McCall (2007).

34 Brand et al. (2012, 109–18), Ong et al. (2008, 171–82), Grossman et al. (2004, 35–43).

35 *Yoga Sūtra of Patañjali,* 1.7.

36 *Yoga Sūtra of Patañjali,* 1.30–1.36.

37 *Yoga Sūtra of Patañjali,* 1.12–1.14.

38 *Yoga Sūtra of Patañjali,* 1.22. These qualities echo gunatraya from the earlier Upanishadic yoga epoch, discussed in chapter 2.

39 Stephens (2010). See chapter 6 for a discussion of the nature and practice of asana.

40 White (2012a).

41 Shusterman (2008 and 2012).

42 Stephens (2012).

43 Todd (1937), Hanna (2004), Lakoff and Johnson (1999).

44 Van der Kolk (2014), Varela et al. (2016).

45 For more on practices of embodiment, see D. H. Johnson (1995), M. Johnson (1995), Macnaughton (2004).

46 An alternative view through the lens of tantra experiences the world more intimately through the senses, what we might call "apratyahara." On tantra's approach to the senses, see Odier (2005) (which includes the ancient *Vijnana Bhairava*). For a Western approach to the value of full sensory experience and consciousness, see Ackerman (1990).

47 Baijal and Srinivasan (2010, 31–38), van Lutterveld et al. (2017, 18–25).

Part II

1 The concept and technique of "playing the edge" was developed by Joel Kramer. Kramer (1977).

Chapter 4

1 Such tension is greater among the elderly and those with other health issues. See Hariprasad et al. (2013, S364–S368), Afonso et al. (2012, 186–93), Kwekkeboom et al. (2010, 126–38), Mustian (2013, 106–15).

2 Several controlled studies validate the effects of yoga on improved sleep. See Chen et al. (2010, 53–61), Chen et al. (2009, 154–63), Innes et al. (2013, 527–35), Yurtkuran et al. (2007, 164–71).

3 In Sanskrit, this pose is named Paschimottanasana, which translates as "Western Stretch Pose," so called for practices that ritually begin by bowing to the east to invite and greet the sun at dawn. Thus, this posture symbolizes the sunset of the practice, folding into a quieter and more reflective space.

4 The Sanskrit name for this pose is Viparita Karani ("Active Reversal").

5 For more on breath-centered meditation, see Kempton (2011).

Chapter 5

1 American Psychological Association (2017).

2 Spielberger et al. (1970), Grillon (2008, 421–37).

3 Emerson (2015).

4 Dating to Wilhelm Reich and William James, there have been many efforts to map physical tension in relation to psychological profiles. A leading example is Keleman (1985).

5 Jacobson (1938). In this edition—unlike the 1929 edition—the title received a subtitle: "A Physiological and Clinical Investigation of Muscular States and Their Significance in Psychology and Medical Practice." The original source on yoga nidra as a defined yoga practice—one that is described using basic yoga concepts and methods in correlation with basic progressive relaxation concepts and methods—is Satyananda Saraswati (1976). Many others have followed, including Miller (2005). Curiously, many yoga nidra authors and teachers refer to the ancient secrets of this entirely modern practice. The only "secret" might be the *khechari mudra* practice in which one gradually snips away the tissue under the base of the tongue to eventually touch the third eye with the tip of the tongue, which is said to lead to yoga nidra. On that claim, see Swatmarama (1985, 310–32). On its connection to yoga nidra, see Swatmarama (1985, 542). Personally, I do not engage in nor recommend any such self-mortification practices and do not believe that anyone must destroy their tissues to have a beneficial yoga practice or healthy life.

6 Luthe (1969), Coué (1922).

Chapter 6

1 Akiskal (1983, 11–20), Qualter et al. (2010, 493–501).

2 Thase et al. (1997, 1009–15).

3 Hofmann et al. (2010, 169–83), Kessler et al. (2001, 289–94), Payne and Crane-Godreau (2015, 71), Walsh and Shapiro (2006, 227–39).

4 Kabat-Zinn (1982, 33–47), Kenny and Williams (2007, 617–25), Kingston et al. (2007, 193–203).

5 Weissman and Weissman (1996).

6 A 2013 review of studies on yoga for psychological problems reveals that most studies are rated as low quality in design and methodology, including studies conducted by the authors of the review. Typical research flaws include very small sample sizes, no double blinding,

high dropout rates, insufficient follow-up, and a tendency among yoga researchers to focus on obscure practices (e.g., Laughter Yoga, SKY Yoga, Silver Yoga, Tibetan Yoga) while not revealing in any detail the specific yoga practices studied. See Balasubramaniam et al. (2013, 1–16). More recent research has improved this picture.

7 Rama (1976), Weintraub (2004), Forbes (2011).

8 Bershadsky et al. (2014, 106–13), Gard et al. (2014, 770), Kinser et al. (2014, 377–83), Kinser et al. (2012, 118–26).

Chapter 7

1 Ohayon et al. (2004, 1255–73).

2 Stores (2009, 85).

3 Stores (2006, 304–38).

4 Stores (2008).

5 Mindell et al. (2006, 1263–76), Gordon et al. (2007, 98–113), Stores (2007, 405–17).

6 Stores (2003, 899–903).

7 Wiggs (2009, 59–62).

8 California Department of Education (2009).

9 Wolfson and Carskadon (2003, 491–506).

10 U.S. Centers for Disease Control and Prevention (2018).

11 Stores (2009, 87). Ironically, Stores first explains that adolescent sleep phase delay is caused by physiological changes, then refers to adolescents' later sleep-wake schedule as an "abnormal sleep pattern" for which he blames the adolescents rather than nature, suggesting chronotherapy, "firm agreement with the adolescent to maintain a new pattern of social activities and sleep," and melatonin in the evening. It is tempting to editorialize here.

12 Gregory and Sadeh (2016, 296–317).

13 Wahlstrom and Owens (2017, 485–90).

14 Touitou (2001, 1083–1100), Swaab et al. (1985, 37–44).

15 Cooke and Ancoli-Israel (2011, 653–65).

16 Ancoli-Israel (1997, 20–30).

17 Vitiello (1996, 284–89).

18 Rediehs et al. (1990, 410–24).

19 Wilcox et al. (2000, 1241–51), Foley et al. (2004, 497–502).

20 Fava (2004, 27–32); Perlis et al. (2006, 104–13), Cole and Dendukuri (2003, 1147–56).

21 Ancoli-Israel and Kripke (1989, 127–32), Blackwell et al. (2006, 405–10).

22 Cooke and Ancoli-Israel (2011, 655–61).

23 Campbell et al. (1988, 141–44), Shochat et al. (2000, 373–80).

Chapter 8

1 Young et al. (1993, 1230–35).

2 Joho et al. (2010, 143–48).

3 Awad et al. (2012, 485–90).

4 Dixon et al. (2005, 1048–54), Peppard and Young (2004, 480–84).

5 Nakayama (1991, 541–55).

6 Clark (2012, 657–67), Lazarus et al. (2003, 199–205), Kletzien et al. (2013, 472–81).

7 Papp (2017, 447–61), Fregosi and Fuller (1997, 295–306), Fuller et al. (1999, 601–13).

8 Swatmarama (1985, 310).

9 Takahashi et al. (2002, 307–13).

10 Sapienza et al. (2011, 21–30).

Chapter 9

1 See chapter 4, endnote 3.

Appendix I

1 American Academy of Sleep Medicine (2014).

Appendix II

1 Stephens (2017, 231–69).

2 Morin et al. (2011, 601–8).

3 Buysse et al. (1989, 193–213).

4 Smets (1995, 315–25).

5 Beck, Steer, and Garbin (1988, 77–100).

6 Beck et al. (1988, 893–97).

7 Spielberger (1983).

8 Ware et al. (1996, 220–33).

Appendix III

1 U.S. National Institutes of Health (2015).

BIBLIOGRAPHY

Abel, G. G., W. D. Murphy, J. V. Becker, and A. Bitar. 1979. "Women's Vaginal Responses during REM Sleep." *Journal of Sex & Marital Therapy* 5: 5–14.

Abrams, Donald I., and Manuel Guzman. 2008. "Cannabinoids and Cancer." In *Integrative Oncology,* edited by Donald I. Abrams and Andrew T. Weil, 246–84. Oxford: Oxford University Press.

Ackerman, Diane. 1990. *A Natural History of the Senses.* New York: Random House.

Afonso, R. F., H. Hachul, E. H. Kozasa, D. Oliveira, V. Goto, D. Rodrigues, S. Tufik, and J. R. Leite. 2012. "Yoga Decreases Insomnia in Postmenopausal Women: A Randomized Clinical Trial." *Menopause* 19: 186–93.

Akerstedt, T., P. Fredlund, M. Gillberg, and B. Jansson. 2002. "Work Load and Work Hours in Relation to Disturbed Sleep and Fatigue in a Large Representative Sample." *Journal of Psychosomatic Research* 53: 585–88.

Akiskal, H. S. 1983. "Dysthymic Disorder: Psychopathology of Proposed Chronic Depressive Subtypes." *American Journal of Psychiatry* 140: 11–20.

American Academy of Sleep Medicine. 2014. *International Classification of Sleep Disorders,* 3rd ed. Darien, IL: American Academy of Sleep Medicine.

American Psychiatric Association. 2013. *Diagnostic and Statistical Manual of Mental Disorders,* 5th ed. (*DSM-V*). Washington, DC: American Psychiatric Association.

American Psychological Association. 2017. *Stress in America: The State of Our Nation.* American Psychological Association. *www.apa.org /images/state-nation_tcm7-225609.pdf.*

Amundsen, A. H., R. Klaeboe, and G. M. Aasvang. 2013. "Long-Term Effects of Noise Reduction Measures on Noise Annoyance and Sleep Disturbance: The Norwegian Facade Insulation Study." *Journal of the Acoustical Society of America* 133: 3921–28.

Amzica, F., A. Nunez, and M. Steriade. 1992. "Delta Frequency (1–4 Hz) Oscillations of Perigeniculate Thalamic Neurons and Their Modulation by Light." *Neuroscience* 51: 285–94.

Ancoli-Israel, S. 1997. "Sleep Problems in Older Adults: Putting Myths to Bed." *Geriatrics* 52 (1): 20–30.

Ancoli-Israel, S., and D. F. Kripke. 1989. "Now I Lay Me Down to Sleep: The Problem of Sleep Fragmentation in Elderly and Demented Residents of Nursing Homes." *Bulletin of Clinical Neurosciences* 54: 127–32.

Andersen, M. L., D. Poyares, and R. S. Alves. 2007. "Sexsomnia: Abnormal Sexual Behavior during Sleep." *Brain Research Review* 56: 271–82.

Arble, D. M., K. M. Ramsey, J. Bass, and F. W. Turek. 2010. "Circadian Disruption and Metabolic Disease: Findings from Animal Models." *Best Practice & Research: Clinical Endocrinology & Metabolism* 24: 785–800.

Aserinsky, E., and N. Kleitman. 1953. "Regularly Occurring Periods of Eye Motility, and Concomitant Phenomena, during Sleep." *Science* 118: 273–74.

Astill, A. G., G. Piantoni, R. J. Raymann, J. C. Vis, J. E. Coppens, M. P. Walker, R. Stickgold, Y. D. Van Der Werf, and E. J. Van Someren. 2014. "Sleep Spindle and Slow Wave Frequency Reflect Motor Skill Performance in Primary School-Age Children." *Frontiers in Human Neuroscience* 8 (November): 910.

Awad, K. M., A. Malhotra, J. H. Barnet, S. F. Quan, and P. E. Peppard. 2012. "Exercise Is Associated with a Reduced Incidence of Sleep-Disordered Breathing." *American Journal of Medicine* 125 (5): 485–90.

Ayas, N. T., D. P. White, and J. E. Manson. 2003. "A Prospective Study of Sleep Duration and Coronary Heart Disease in Women." *Archives of Internal Medicine* 163: 205–9.

Babson, K. A., and M. T. Feldner. 2010. "Temporal Relations between Sleep Problems and Both Traumatic Event Exposure and PTSD: A Critical Review of the Empirical Literature." *Journal of Anxiety Disorders* 24 (1): 1–15.

Backes, Michael. 2014. *Cannabis Pharmacy: The Practical Guide to Medical Marijuana.* New York: Black Dog & Leventhal.

Baijal, S., and N. Srinivasan. 2010. "Theta Activity and Meditative States: Spectral Changes during Concentrative Meditation." *Cognitive Processing* 11: 31–38.

Balasubramaniam, M., S. Telles, and P. M. Doraiswamy. 2013. "Yoga on Our Minds: A Systematic Review of Yoga for Neuropsychiatric Disorders." *Frontiers in Psychiatry* 3 (117): 1–16.

Barger, L. K., B. E. Cade, and N. T. Ayas. 2005. "Extended Work Shifts and the Risk of Motor Vehicle Crashes among Interns." *New England Journal of Medicine* 352: 15–34.

Basheer, R., R. E. Strecker, M. M. Thakkar, and R. W. McCarley. 2004. "Adenosine and Sleep-Wake Regulation." *Progress in Neurobiology* 73: 379–96.

Bchir, F., M. Dogui, R. Ben Fradj, M. J. Arnaud, and S. Saguem. 2006. "Differences in Pharmacokinetic and Electroencephalographic Responses to Caffeine in Sleep-Sensitive and Non-sensitive Subjects." *Comptes Rendus Biologies* 329 (7): 512–19.

Beck, A. T. 1975. *Cognitive Therapy and the Emotional Disorders.* Madison, CT: International Universities Press.

Beck, A. T., N. Epstein, G. Brown, and R. A. Steer. 1988. "An Inventory for Measuring Clinical Anxiety: Psychometric Properties." *Journal of Consulting and Clinical Psychology* 56: 893–97.

Beck, A. T., R. A. Steer, and M. G. Garbin. 1988. "Psychometric Properties of the Beck Depression Inventory: Twenty-Five Years of Evaluation." *Clinical Psychology Review* 8: 77–100.

Beers, T. 2000. "Flexible Schedules and Shift Work: Replacing the '9-to-5' Workday?" *Monthly Labor Review* 23: 33–40.

Bélanger, L., A. G. Harvey, É. Fortier-Brochu, et al. 2016. "Impact of Comorbid Anxiety and Depressive Disorders on Treatment Response to Cognitive Behavior Therapy for Insomnia." *Journal of Consulting and Clinical Psychology* 84: 659–67.

Belleville, G., S. Guay, and A. Marchand. 2011. "Persistence of Sleep Disturbances Following Cognitive-Behavior Therapy for Posttraumatic Stress Disorder." *Journal of Psychosomatic Research* 70 (4): 318–27.

Benowitz, N. L. 1990. "Clinical Pharmacology of Caffeine." *Annual Review of Medicine* 41: 277–88.

Bernert, R. A., and T. E. Joiner. 2007. "Sleep Disturbances and Suicide Risk: A Review of the Literature." *Neuropsychiatric Disease and Treatment* 3: 735–43.

Bershadsky, S. L., L. Trumpfheller, H. B. Kimble, D. Pipaloff, and I. S. Yim. 2014. "The Effect of Prenatal Hatha Yoga on Affect, Cortisol and Depressive Symptoms." *Complementary Therapies in Clinical Practice* 20 (2): 106–13.

Bes, F., H. Schulz, Y. Navelet, and P. Salzarulo. 1991. "The Distribution of Slow-Wave Sleep across the Night: A Comparison for Infants, Children, and Adults." *Sleep* 14: 5–12.

Besedovsky, L., T. Lange, and J. Born. 2012. "Sleep and Immune Function." *Pflugers Archives* 463: 121–37.

Bhaskar, S., D. Hemavathy, and S. Prasad. 2016. "Prevalence of Chronic Insomnia in Adult Patients and Its Correlation with Medical Comorbidities." *Journal of Family Medicine and Primary Care* 5 (4): 780–84.

Blackwell, T., K. Yaffe, S. Ancoli-Israel, J. L. Schneider, J. A. Cauley, T. A. Hillier, H. A. Fink, and K. L. Stone. 2006. "Poor Sleep Is Associated with Impaired Cognitive Function in Older Women: The Study of Osteoporotic Fractures." *Journal of Gerontology: Medical Sciences* 61 (4): 405–10.

Blanco, M., N. Krober, and D. P. Cardinali. 2004. "A Survey of Sleeping Difficulties in an Urban Latin American Population." *Review of Neurology* 39 (2): 155–59.

Blavatsky, Helena Petrovna. 1933. *The Secret Doctrine,* vol. II. Wheaton, IL: Theosophical Publishing House.

Blessing, E. M., M. M. Steenkamp, J. Manzanares, and C. R. Marmar. 2015. "Cannabidiol as a Potential Treatment for Anxiety Disorders." *Neurotherapeutics* 12 (4): 825–36.

Bonnet, M. H., and D. L. Arand. 2010. "Hyperarousal and Insomnia: State of the Science." *Sleep Medicine Review* 14: 9–15.

Borbély, A. A. 1982. "A Two Process Model of Sleep Regulation." *Human Neurobiology* 1 (3): 195–204.

Borbély, A. A., and P. Achermann. 1999. "Sleep Homeostasis and Models of Sleep Regulation." *Journal of Biological Rhythms* 14: 557–68.

Borbély, A. A., S. Daan, A. Wirz-Justice, and T. Deboer. 2016. "The Two-Process Model of Sleep Regulation: A Reappraisal." *Journal of Sleep Research* 25: 131–43.

Born, J., and I. Wilhelm. 2012. "System Consolidation of Memory during Sleep." *Psychological Research* 76: 192–203.

Boutrel, B., and G. F. Koob. 2004. "What Keeps Us Awake: The Neuropharmacology of Stimulants and Wakefulness-Promoting Medications." *Sleep* 27: 1181–94.

Brand, S., and E. Holsboer-Trachsler, J. R. Naranjo, and S. Schmidt. 2012. "Influence of Mindfulness Practice on Cortisol and Sleep in Long-Term and Short-Term Meditators." *Neuropsychobiology* 65: 109–18.

Brooks, E., and M. M. Canal. 2013. "Development of Circadian Rhythms: Role of Postnatal Light Environment." *Neuroscience and Biobehavioral Reviews* 37 (4): 551–60.

Brown, R. E., R. Basheer, J. T. McKenna, R. E. Strecker, and R. W. McCarley. 2012. "Control of Sleep and Wakefulness." *Physiological Review* 92 (3): 1088.

Brown, R. E., and J. T. McKenna. 2015. "Turning a Negative into a Positive: Ascending GABAergic Control of Cortical Activation and Arousal." *Frontiers of Neurology* 6: 135.

Budnick, L. D., S. E. Lerman, T. L. Baker, H. Jones, and C. A. Czeisler. 1994. "Sleep and Alertness in a 12-Hour Rotating Shift Work Environment." *Journal of Occupational Medicine* 36: 1295–300.

Buxton, O. M., and E. Marcelli. 2010. "Short and Long Sleep Are Positively Associated with Obesity, Diabetes, Hypertension, and Cardiovascular Disease among Adults in the United States." *Social Science & Medicine* 71: 1027–36.

Buysse, D. J. 2014. "Sleep Health: Can We Define It? Does It Matter?" *Sleep* 37: 9–17.

Buysse, D. J., C. F. Reynolds 3rd, T. H. Monk, S. R. Berman, and D. J. Kupfer. 1989. "The Pittsburgh Sleep Quality Index: A New Instrument for Psychiatric Practice and Research." *Psychiatry Research* 28 (2): 193–213.

Buzsáki, G. 1989. "Two-Stage Model of Memory Trace Formation: A Role for 'Noisy' Brain States." *Neuroscience* 31: 551–70.

Buzsáki, G., and A. Draguhn. 2004. "Neuronal Oscillations in Cortical Networks." *Science* 304: 1926–29.

California Department of Education. 2009. *Physical Education Framework for California Public Schools: Kindergarten through Grade Twelve.* Sacramento, CA: California Department of Education.

Campbell, S. S., D. F. Kripke, J. C. Gillin, and J. C. Hrubovcak. 1988. "Exposure to Light in Healthy Elderly Subjects and Alzheimer's Patients." *Physiology and Behavior* 42: 141–44.

Cappuccio, F. P., D. Cooper, L. D'Elia, P. Strazzullo, and M. A. Miller. 2011. "Sleep Duration Predicts Cardiovascular Outcomes: A Systematic Review and Meta-analysis of Prospective Studies." *European Heart Journal* 32: 1484–92.

Cappuccio, F. P., F. M. Taggart, N. B. Kandala, A. Currie, E. Peile, S. Stranges, and M. A. Miller. 2008. "Meta-analysis of Short Sleep Duration and Obesity in Children and Adults." *Sleep* 31: 619–26.

Carskadon, M. A. 2011. "Sleep in Adolescents: The Perfect Storm." *Pediatric Clinics of North America* 58 (3): 637–47.

Chen, K. M., M. H. Chen, and H. C. Chao. 2009. "Sleep Quality, Depression State, and Health Status of Older Adults after Silver Yoga Exercises: Cluster Randomized Trial." *International Journal of Nursing Studies* 46: 154–63.

Chen, K. M., M. H. Chen, and M. H. Lin. 2010. "Effects of Yoga on Sleep Quality and Depression in Elders in Assisted Living Facilities." *Journal of Nursing Research* 18: 53–61.

Chennaoui, M., F. Sauvet, C. Drogou, P. Van Beers, and C. Langrume. 2011. "Effect of One Night of Sleep Loss on Changes in Tumor Necrosis Factor Alpha (TNF-α) Levels in Healthy Men." *Cytokine* 56: 318–24.

Chong, Y., C. D. Fryar, and Q. Gu. 2013. "Prescription Sleep Aid Use among Adults: United States, 2005–2010." NCHS data brief, no. 127. Hyattsville, MD: National Center for Health Statistics.

Clark, H. M. 2012. "Specificity of Training in the Lingual Musculature." *Journal of Speech, Language, and Hearing Research* 55: 657–67.

Cohen, S., W. J. Doyle, C. M. Alper, D. Janicki-Deverts, and R. B. Turner. 2009. "Sleep Habits and Susceptibility to the Common Cold." *Archives of Internal Medicine* 169: 62–67.

Cole, M. G., and N. Dendukuri. 2003. "Risk Factors for Depression among Elderly Community Subjects: A Systematic Review and Meta-analysis." *American Journal of Psychiatry* 160 (6): 1147–56.

Cole, S. W. 2009. "Chronic Inflammation and Breast Cancer Recurrence." *Journal of Clinical Oncology* 27: 3418–19.

Conlon, M., N. Lightfoot, and N. Kreiger. 2007. "Rotating Shift Work and Risk of Prostate Cancer." *Epidemiology* 18: 182–83.

Cooke, J., and S. Ancoli-Israel. 2011. "Normal and Abnormal Sleep in the Elderly." *Handbook of Clinical Neurology* 98: 653–65.

Cota, D., M. H. Tschop, T. L. Horvath, and A. S. Levine. 2006. "Cannabinoids, Opioids and Eating Behavior: The Molecular Face of Hedonism?" *Brain Research Review* 51: 85–107.

Coué, Émile. 1922. *Self Mastery through Conscious Autosuggestion.* Translated by Archibald S. Van Orden. New York: Malkan.

Czeisler, C. A. 1995. "The Effect of Light on the Human Circadian Pacemaker." *Ciba Foundation Symposium* 183: 254–302.

Daly, J. W., and B. B. Fredholm. 1998. "Caffeine: An Atypical Drug of Dependence." *Drug and Alcohol Dependency* 51 (1–2): 199–206.

Dement, W., and N. Kleitman. 1957a. "Cyclic Variations in EEG during Sleep and Their Relation to Eye Movements, Body Motility, and Dreaming." *Electroencephalography and Clinical Neurophysiology,* Suppl. 9: 673–90.

Dement, W., and N. Kleitman. 1957b. "The Relation of Eye Movements during Sleep to Dream Activity: An Objective Method for the Study of Dreaming." *Journal of Experimental Psychology* 53 (5): 339–46.

Descartes, René. 1993. *Meditations on First Philosophy.* Translated by Donald A. Cress. Indianapolis: Hackett.

Dew, M. A., C. C. Hoch, D. J. Buysse, T. H. Monk, and A. E. Begley. 2003. "Healthy Older Adults' Sleep Predicts All-Cause Mortality at 4 to 19 Years of Follow-up." *Psychosomatic Medicine* 65: 63–73.

Diekelmann, J., and J. Born. 2010. "The Memory Function of Sleep." *National Review of Neuroscience* 11: 114–26.

Dinges, D. F., F. Pack, K. Williams, K. A. Gillen, J. W. Powell, G. E. Ott, C. Aptowicz, and A. I. Pack. 1997. "Cumulative Sleepiness, Mood Disturbance, and Psychomotor Vigilance Performance Decrements during a Week of Sleep Restricted to 4–5 Hours per Night." *Sleep* 20: 267–77.

Dixon, J. B., L. M. Schachter, and P. E. O'Brien. 2005. "Polysomnography before and after Weight Loss in Obese Patients with Severe Sleep Apnea." *International Journal of Obesity* (London) 29 (9): 1048–54.

Domhoff, G. William. 2018. *The Emergence of Dreaming: Mind-Wandering, Embodied Simulation, and the Default Network.* New York: Oxford University Press.

Drake, C., T. Roehrs, J. Shambroom, and T. Roth. 2013. "Caffeine Effects on Sleep Taken 0, 3, or 6 Hours before Going to Bed." *Journal of Clinical Sleep Medicine* 9: 1195–200.

Driver, H. S., G. G. Rogers, and D. Mitchell. 1994. "Prolonged Endurance Exercise and Sleep Disruption." *Medicine & Science in Sports & Exercise* 26: 903–7.

Dubessy, A. L., S. Leu-Semenescu, V. Attali, J. B. Maranci, and I. Arnulf. 2017. "Sexsomnia: A Specialized Non-REM Parasomnia?" *Sleep* 40 (2) (February 1).

Duffy, J. F., D. J. Dijk, and E. B. Klerman. 1998. "Later Endogenous Circadian Temperature Nadir relative to an Earlier Wake Time in Older People." *American Journal of Physiology* 275: R1478–R1487.

300   YOGA FOR BETTER SLEEP

Dunwiddie, T. V., and S. A. Masino. 2001. "The Role and Regulation of Adenosine in the Central Nervous System." *Annual Review of Neuroscience* 24: 31–55.

Ebrahim, I. O., C. M. Shapiro, A. J. Williams, and P. B. Fenwick. 2013. "Alcohol and Sleep I: Effects on Normal Sleep." *Alcoholism: Clinical and Experimental Research* 37: 539–49.

Ekbom, K., and J. Ulfberg. 2009. "Restless Legs Syndrome." *Journal of Internal Medicine* 266: 419–31.

Elklit, A., P. Hyland, and M. Shevlin. 2014. "Evidence of Symptom Profiles Consistent with Posttraumatic Stress Disorder and Complex Posttraumatic Stress Disorder in Different Trauma Samples." *European Journal of Psychotraumatology* 5 (1).

Ellenbogen, J. M. 2005. "Cognitive Benefits of Sleep and Their Loss due to Sleep Deprivation." *Neurology* 64: E25–E27.

Emerson, David. 2015. *Trauma-Sensitive Yoga: Bringing the Body into Treatment*. New York: W. W. Norton.

Engeda, J., B. Mezuk, S. Ratliff, and Y. Ning. 2013. "Association between Duration and Quality of Sleep and the Risk of Pre-diabetes: Evidence from NHANES." *Diabetes Medicine* 30: 676–80.

Fancher, Robert T. 1995. *Cultures of Healing: Correcting the Image of American Mental Health Care*. New York: W. W. Freeman.

Fava, M. 2004. "Daytime Sleepiness and Insomnia as Correlates of Depression." *Journal of Clinical Psychiatry* 65 (Suppl. 16): 27–32.

Fernandez-Mendoza, J., A. N. Vgontzas, D. Liao, M. L. Shaffer, and A. Vela-Bueno. 2012. "Insomnia with Objective Short Sleep Duration and Incident Hypertension: The Penn State Cohort." *Hypertension* 60 (4): 929–35.

Finan, P. H., B. R. Goodin, and M. T. Smith. 2013. "The Association of Sleep and Pain: An Update and a Path Forward." *Journal of Pain* 14: 1539–52.

Flausino, N. H., J. M. Da Silva Prado, S. S. de Queiroz, S. Tufik, and M. T. de Mello. 2012. "Physical Exercise Performed before Bedtime Improves the Sleep Pattern of Healthy Young Good Sleepers." *Psychophysiology* 49: 186–92.

Foley, D. J., S. Ancoli-Israel, P. Britz, and J. Walsh. 2004. "Sleep Disturbances and Chronic Disease in Older Adults: Results of the 2003 National Sleep Foundation Sleep in America Survey." *Journal of Psychosomatic Research* 56 (5): 497–502.

Folkard, S. 1989. "Shift Work: A Growing Occupational Hazard." *Occupational Medicine* (London) 41: 182–86.

Folkard, S., and T. Åkersted. 2004. "Trends in the Risk of Accidents and Injuries and Their Implications for Models of Fatigue and Performance." *Aviation, Space, and Environmental Medicine* 75: A161–A167.

Forbes, Bo. 2011. *Yoga for Emotional Balance: Simple Practices to Help Relieve Anxiety and Depression*. Boston: Shambhala.

Ford, D. E., and D. B. Kamerow. 1989. "Epidemiologic Study of Sleep Disturbances and Psychiatric Disorders: An Opportunity for Prevention?" *Journal of the American Medical Association* 262: 1479–84.

Foulkes, D., and G. W. Domhoff. 2014. "Bottom-up or Top-down in Dream Neuroscience? A Top-down Critique of Two Bottom-up Studies." *Consciousness and Cognition* 27: 168–71.

Fowler, P. M., W. Knez, S. C. Crowcroft, A. E. Mendham, J. Miller, and C. Sargent. 2017. "Greater Effect of East versus West Travel on Jet Lag, Sleep, and Team Sport Performance." *Medicine & Science in Sports & Exercise* 49: 2548–61.

Frary, C. D., R. K. Johnson, and M. Q. Wang. 2005. "Food Sources and Intakes of Caffeine in the Diets of Persons in the United States." *Journal of the American Dietary Association* 105 (1): 110–13.

Freedman, R. R., and T. A. Roehrs. 2007. "Sleep Disturbance in Menopause." *Menopause* 14 (5): 826–29.

Fregosi, R., and D. Fuller. 1997. "Respiratory-Related Control of Extrinsic Tongue Muscle Activity." *Respiratory Physiology* 110: 295–306.

Freud, Sigmund. 1994 (1899). *The Interpretation of Dreams*. New York: Modern Library.

Fulda, S., and H. Schulz. 2001. "Cognitive Dysfunction in Sleep Disorders." *Sleep Medicine Review* 5: 423–45.

Fuller, D., J. Williams, P. Janssen, and R. Fregosi. 1999. "Effect of Coactivation of Tongue Protrudor and Retractor Muscles on Tongue Movements and Pharyngeal Airflow Mechanics in the Rat." *Journal of Physiology* (London) 519: 601–13.

Gangwisch, J. E. 2009. "Epidemiological Evidence for the Links between Sleep, Circadian Rhythms and Metabolism." *Obesity Review* 10 (Suppl. 2): 37–45.

Gangwisch, J. E., D. Malaspina, B. Boden-Albala, and S. B. Heymsfield. 2005. "Inadequate Sleep as a Risk Factor for Obesity: Analyses of the NHANES I." *Sleep* 28: 1289–96.

Gangwisch, J. E., D. Malaspina, K. Posner, L. A. Babiss, S. B. Heymsfield, J. B. Turner, G. K. Zammit, and T. G. Pickering. 2010. "Insomnia and Sleep Duration as Mediators of the Relationship between Depression and Hypertension Incidence." *American Journal of Hypertension* 23: 62–69.

Gaoni, Y., and R. Mechoulam. 1964. "Isolation, Structure, and Partial Synthesis of an Active Constituent of Hashish." *Journal of the American Chemistry Society* 86: 1646–47.

Gard, T., J. J. Noggle, C. L. Park, D. R. Vago, and A. Wilson. 2014. "Potential Self-Regulatory Mechanisms of Yoga for Psychological Health." *Frontiers in Human Neuroscience* 8: 770.

Gautier-Sauvigné, S., D. Colas, P. Parmantier, P. Clement, A. Gharib, N. Sarda, and R. Cespuglio. 2005. "Nitric Oxide and Sleep." *Sleep Medicine Review* 9: 101–13.

Gehrman, P. R., and G. C. Harb. 2010. "Treatment of Nightmares in the Context of Posttraumatic Stress Disorder." *Journal of Clinical Psychology* 66: 1185–94.

Germain, A. 2013. "Sleep Disturbances as the Hallmark of PTSD: Where Are We Now?" *American Journal of Psychiatry* 170 (4): 372–82.

Glovinsky, Paul, and Arthur Spielman. 2006. *The Insomnia Answer.* New York: Penguin Group.

Glovinsky, Paul, and Arthur Spielman. 2017. *You Are Getting Sleepy: Lifestyle-Based Solutions for Insomnia.* New York: Diversion Books.

Goldstein-Piekarski, A. N., S. M. Greer, J. M. Saletin, and M. P. Walker. 2015. "Sleep Deprivation Impairs the Human Central and Peripheral Nervous System Discrimination of Social Threat." *Journal of Neuroscience* 35 (28): 10135–45.

Gordon, J., N. J. King, E. Gullone, P. Muris, and T. H. Ollendick. 2007. "Treatment of Children's Nighttime Fears: The Need for a Modern Randomized Controlled Trial." *Clinical Psychology Review* 27: 98–113.

Gregory, A. M., and A. Sadeh. 2016. "Annual Research Review: Sleep Problems in Childhood Psychiatric Disorders—A Review of the Latest Science." *Journal of Child Psychology and Psychiatry* 57 (3): 296–317.

Griefahn, B., P. Brode, A. Marks, and M. Basner. 2008. "Autonomic Arousals related to Traffic Noise during Sleep." *Sleep* 31: 569–77.

Grillon, C. 2008. "Models and Mechanisms of Anxiety: Evidence from Startle Studies." *Psychopharmacology* 199: 421–37.

Grossman, P., L. Niemann, S. Schmidt, and H. Walach. 2004. "Mindfulness-Based Stress Reduction and Health Benefits: A Meta-analysis." *Journal of Psychosomatic Research* 57: 35–43.

Gubin, D. G., D. Weinert., S. V. Rybina, L. A. Danilova, S. V. Solovieva, A. M. Durov, N. Y. Prokopiev, and P. A. Ushakov. 2017. "Activity, Sleep and Ambient Light Have a Different Impact on Circadian Blood Pressure, Heart Rate and Body Temperature Rhythms." *Chronobiology International* 34 (5): 632–49.

Gujar, N., S. S. Yoo, P. Hu, and M. P. Walker. 2010. "The Unrested Resting Brain: Sleep Deprivation Alters Activity within the Default-Mode Network." *Journal of Cognitive Neuroscience* 22: 1637–48.

Gyatso, Khedrup Norsang. 2004. *Ornament of Stainless Light.* Translated by Gavin Kilty. The Library of Tibetan Classics 14. Boston: Wisdom Publications.

Hall, M., R. Vasko, and D. J. Buysse. 2004. "Acute Stress Affects Heart Rate Variability during Sleep." *Psychosomatic Medicine* 66: 56–62.

Hall Brown, T., and T. A. Mellman. 2014. "The Influence of PTSD, Sleep Fears, and Neighborhood Stress on Insomnia and Short Sleep Duration in Urban, Young Adult, African Americans." *Behavioral Sleep Medicine* 12 (3): 198–206.

Hanna, Thomas. 2004. *Somatics: Reawakening the Mind's Control of Movement, Flexibility, and Health.* Cambridge, MA: Da Capo Press.

Hansen, M., I. Janssen, A. Schiff, P. C. Zee, and M. L. Dubocovich. 2005. "The Impact of School Daily Schedule on Adolescent Sleep." *Pediatrics* 115 (6): 1555–61.

Hariprasad, V. R., P. T. Sivakumar, V. Koparde, S. Varambally, J. Thirthalli, and M. Varghese. 2013. "Effect of Yoga Intervention on Sleep and Quality-of-Life in Elderly: A Randomized Controlled Trial." *Indian Journal of Psychiatry* 55: S364–S368.

Harvey, A. G. 2000. "Sleep Hygiene and Sleep-Onset Insomnia." *Journal of Nervous and Mental Disease* 188: 53–55.

Harvey, A. G. 2001. "Insomnia: Symptom or Diagnosis?" *Clinical Psychology Review* 21 (7): 1037–59.

Harvey, A. G., A. M. Soehner, and K. A. Kaplan. 2015. "Treating Insomnia Improves Mood State, Sleep, and Functioning in Bipolar Disorder: A Pilot Randomized Controlled Trial." *Journal of Consulting and Clinical Psychology* 83 (3): 564–77.

Haskell, C. F., D. O. Kennedy, K. A. Wesnes, and A. B. Scholey. 2005. "Cognitive and Mood Improvements of Caffeine in Habitual Consumers and Habitual Non-consumers of Caffeine." *Psychopharmacology* (Berlin) 179 (4) (June): 813–25.

Hasler, G., D. J. Buysse, R. Klaghofer, A. Gamma, V. Ajdacic, D. Eich, W. Rossler, and J. Angst. 2004. "The Association between Short Sleep Duration and Obesity in Young Adults: A 13-Year Prospective Study." *Sleep* 27 (4): 661–66.

Haus, E. L., and M. H. Smolensky. 2013. "Shift Work and Cancer Risk: Potential Mechanistic Roles of Circadian Disruption, Light at Night, and Sleep Deprivation." *Sleep Medicine Review* 17: 273–84.

Hayaishi, O., Y. Urade, N. Eguchi, and Z. L. Huang. 2004. "Genes for Prostaglandin D Synthase and Receptor as Well as Adenosine A2A Receptor Are Involved in the Homeostatic Regulation of NREM Sleep." *Archives Italiennes de Biologie* 142: 533–39.

Heslop, P., G. D. Smith, C. Metcalfe, J. Macleod, and C. Hart. 2002. "Sleep Duration and Mortality: The Effect of Short or Long Sleep Duration on Cardiovascular and All-Cause Mortality in Working Men and Women." *Sleep Medicine* 3: 305–14.

Hirshkowitz, M., and M. H. Schmidt. 2005. "Sleep-Related Erections: Clinical Perspectives of Neural Mechanisms." *Sleep Medicine Review* 9: 311–29.

Hobson, J. A., R. W. McCarley, and P. W. Wyzinski. 1975. "Sleep Cycle Oscillation: Reciprocal Discharge by Two Brainstem Neuronal Groups." *Science* 189: 55–58.

Hofmann, S. G., A. T. Sawyer, A. A. Witt, and D. Oh. 2010. "The Effect of Mindfulness-Based Therapy on Anxiety and Depression: A Meta-analytic Review." *Journal of Consulting and Clinical Psychology* 78 (2): 169–83.

Huang, Z. L., Y. Urade, and O. Hayaishi. 2007. "Prostaglandins and Adenosine in the Regulation of Sleep and Wakefulness." *Current Opinion in Pharmacology* 7: 33–38.

Imeri, L., and M. R. Opp. 2009. "How (and Why) the Immune System Makes Us Sleep." *Nature Reviews Neuroscience* 10: 199–210.

Innes, K. E., T. K. Selfe, P. Agarwal, K. Williams, and K. L. Flack. 2013. "Efficacy of an Eight-Week Yoga Intervention on Symptoms of Restless Legs Syndrome (RLS): A Pilot Study." *Journal of Alternative and Complementary Medicine* 19 (6): 527–35.

Jacobs, B. L., and E. C. Azmitia. 1992. "Structure and Function of the Brain Serotonin System." *Physiological Review* 72: 165–229.

Jacobs, Gregg. 1998. *Say Goodnight to Insomnia.* New York: Henry Holt.

Jacobson, Edmund. 1938. *Progressive Relaxation.* Chicago: University of Chicago Press.

Johnson, Don Hanlon, ed. 1995. *Bone, Breath, and Gesture: Practices of Embodiment.* Berkeley, CA: North Atlantic Books.

Johnson, Mark. 1995. *The Body in the Mind: The Bodily Basis of Meaning, Imagination, and Reason.* Chicago: University of Chicago Press.

Joho, S., Y. Oda, and T. Hirai. 2010. "Impact of Sleeping Position on Central Sleep Apnea/Cheyne-Stokes Respiration in Patients with Heart Failure." *Sleep Medicine* 11: 143–48.

Jones, B. E. 1993. "The Organization of Central Cholinergic Systems and Their Functional Importance in Sleep-Waking States." *Progress in Brain Research* 98: 61–71.

Jones, B. E. 2003. "Arousal Systems." *Frontiers in Bioscience* 8: 438–51.

Jones, B. E. 2005. "Basic Mechanisms of Sleep-Wake States." In *Principles and Practices of Sleep Medicine,* 4th ed., edited by M. Kryger, T. Roth, and W. Dement, 136–53. Philadelphia: Elsevier Saunders.

Jouvet, M. 1962. "Recherches sur les structures nerveuses et les mécanismes responsables des différentes phases du sommeil physiologique." *Archives Italiennes de Biologie* 100: 125–206.

Jung, Carl. 2002. *Dreams.* New York: Routledge.

Kabat-Zinn, Jon. 1982. "An Outpatient Program in Behavioral Medicine for Chronic Pain Patients based on the Practice of Mindfulness Meditation: Theoretical Considerations and Preliminary Results." *General Hospital Psychiatry* 4: 33–47.

Kahana, M. J. 2006. "The Cognitive Correlates of Human Brain Oscillations." *Journal of Neuroscience* 26: 1669–72.

Kaida, K., K. Niki, and J. Born. 2015. "Role of Sleep for Encoding of Emotional Memory." *Neurobiology of Learning and Memory* 121: 72–79.

Kales, J. D., A. Kales, and C. R. Soldatos. 1980. "Night Terrors: Clinical Characteristics and Personality Patterns." *Archives of General Psychiatry* 37: 1413–17.

Kamphuis, J., P. Meerlo, J. M. Koolhaas, and M. Lancel. 2012. "Poor Sleep as a Potential Causal Factor in Aggression and Violence." *Sleep Medicine* 13: 327–34.

Katz, I., J. Stradling, A. S. Slutsky, N. Zamel, and V. Hoffstein. 1990. "Do Patients with Obstructive Sleep Apnea Have Thick Necks?" *American Review of Respiratory Disease* 141 (5, Part 1): 1228–31.

Kawakami, N., N. Takatsuka, and H. Shimizu. 2004. "Sleep Disturbance and Onset of Type 2 Diabetes." *Diabetes Care* 27: 282–83.

Keleman, Stanley. 1985. *Emotional Anatomy: The Structure of Experience.* Berkeley, CA: Center Press.

Kempton, Sally. 2011. *Meditation for the Love of It: Enjoying Your Own Deepest Experience.* Boulder, CO: Sounds True.

Kempton, Sally. 2013. *Awakening Shakti: The Transformative Power of the Goddesses of Yoga.* Boulder, CO: Sounds True.

Kempton, Sally. 2014. *Awakening to Kali: The Goddess of Radical Transformation.* Boulder, CO: Sounds True.

Kenny, M. A., and J. M. G. Williams. 2007. "Treatment-Resistant Depressed Patients Show a Good Response to Mindfulness-Based Cognitive Therapy." *Behaviour Research and Therapy* 45: 617–25.

Kessler, R. C., J. Soukup, and R. B. Davi. 2001. "The Use of Complementary and Alternative Therapies to Treat Anxiety and Depression in the United States." *American Journal of Psychiatry* 158 (2): 289–94.

Khalsa, S. B., J. E. Jewett, C. Cajochen, and C. A. Czeisler. 2003. "A Phase Response Curve to Single Bright Light Pulses in Human Subjects." *Journal of Physiology* 549: 945–52.

Khalsa, S. B., T. McCall, S. Telles, and L. Cohen. 2016. *The Principles and Practice of Yoga in Health Care.* London: Handspring.

Killgore, W. D. 2010. "Effects of Sleep Deprivation on Cognition." *Progress in Brain Research.* 185: 105–29.

Kingston, T., B. Dooley, A. Bates, E. Lawlor, and K. Malone. 2007. "Mindfulness-Based Cognitive Therapy for Residual Depressive Symptoms." *Psychology and Psychotherapy: Theory, Research and Practice* 80: 193–203.

Kinser, P. A., R. K. Elswick, and S. Kornstein. 2014. "Potential Long-Term Effects of a Mind-Body Intervention for Women with Major Depressive Disorder: Sustained Mental Health Improvements with a Pilot Yoga Intervention." *Archives of Psychiatric Nursing* 28 (6): 377–83.

Kinser, P. A., L. Goehler, and A. G. Taylor. 2012. "How Might Yoga Help Depression? A Neurobiological Perspective." *Explore* 8 (2): 118–26.

Kletzien, H., J. A. Russell, G. E. Leverson, and N. P. Connor. 2013. "Differential Effects of Targeted Tongue Exercise and Treadmill Running on

Aging Tongue Muscle Structure and Contractile Properties." *Journal of Applied Physiology* 114 (4): 472–81.

Knutsson, A. 2003. "Health Disorders of Shift Workers." *Occupational Medicine* (London) 53: 103–8.

Kramer, Joel. 1977. "A New Look at Yoga." *Yoga Journal,* January.

Krause, A. J., E. B. Simon, B. A. Mander, S. M. Greer, J. M. Saletin, A. N. Goldstein-Piekarski, and M. P. Walker. 2017. "The Sleep-Deprived Human Brain." *Nature Reviews Neuroscience* 18 (7): 404–18.

Kronholm, E., T. Laatikainen, M. Peltonen, R. Sippola, and T. Partonen. 2011. "Self-Reported Sleep Duration, All-Cause Mortality, Cardiovascular Mortality and Morbidity in Finland." *Sleep Medicine* 12: 215–21.

Kubo, T., I. Oyama, T. Nakamura, K. Shirane, and H. Otsuka. 2011. "Retrospective Cohort Study of the Risk of Obesity among Shift Workers: Findings from the Industry-Based Shift Workers' Health Study, Japan." *Occupational and Environmental Medicine* 68: 327–31.

Kurien, P. A., S. Y. Chong, L. J. Ptáček, and Y. H. Fu. 2013. "Sick and Tired: How Molecular Regulators of Human Sleep Schedules and Duration Impact Immune Function." *Current Opinion in Neurobiology* 23 (5): 873–79.

Kuriyama, K., R. Stickgold, and M. P. Walker. 2004. "Sleep-Dependent Learning and Motor Skill Complexity." *Learning & Memory* 11: 705–13.

Kurlansik, S. L., and A. D. Ibay. 2012. "Seasonal Affective Disorder." *American Family Physician* 86 (11) (December 1): 1037–41.

Kurth, S., M. Ringli, A. Geiger, M. LeBourgeois, O. G. Jenni, and R. Huber. 2010. "Mapping of Cortical Activity in the First Two Decades of Life: A High-Density Sleep Electroencephalogram Study." *Journal of Neuroscience* 30: 13211–19.

Kwekkeboom, K. L., C. H. Cherwin, J. W. Lee, and B. Wanta. 2010. "Mind-Body Treatments for the Pain-Fatigue-Sleep Disturbance Symptom Cluster in Persons with Cancer." *Journal of Pain and Symptom Management* 39: 126–38.

Lack, L. C., M. Bailey, N. Lovato, and H. Wright. 2009. "Chronotype Differences in Circadian Rhythms of Temperature, Melatonin, and Sleepiness as Measured in a Modified Constant Routine Protocol." *Nature and Science of Sleep* 1: 1–8.

Lack, L. C., M. Gradisar, E. J. Van Someren, H. R. Wright, and K. Lushington. 2008. "The Relationship between Insomnia and Body Temperature." *Sleep Medicine Review* 12: 307–17.

Lakoff, George, and Mark Johnson. 1999. *Philosophy in the Flesh: The Embodied Mind and Its Challenge to Western Thought.* New York: Basic Books.

Lange, T., S. Dimitrov, and J. Born. 2010. "Effects of Sleep and Circadian Rhythm on the Human Immune System." *Annals of the New York Academy of Sciences* 1193: 48–59.

Lazarus, C., J. Logemann, C. Huang, and A. Rademaker. 2003. "Effects of Two Types of Tongue Strengthening Exercises in Young Normals." *Folia Phoniatrica et Logopaedica* 55: 199–205.

Leger, D., B. Poursain, D. Neubauer, and M. Uchiyama. 2008. "An International Survey of Sleeping Problems in the General Population." *Current Medical Research and Opinion* 24: 307–17.

Lin, J. S. 2000. "Brain Structures and Mechanisms Involved in the Control of Cortical Activation and Wakefulness, with Emphasis on the Posterior Hypothalamus and Histaminergic Neurons." *Sleep Medicine Review* 4: 471–503.

LoBello, S. G., and S. Mehta. 2018. "No Evidence of Seasonal Variation in Mild Forms of Depression." *Journal of Behavioral Therapy and Experimental Psychiatry* 62 (September 15): 72–79.

Lokhorst, Gert-Jan. 2017. "Descartes and the Pineal Gland." In *Stanford Encyclopedia of Philosophy* (Winter 2017), edited by Edward N. Zalta. *https://plato.stanford.edu/archives/win2017/entries/pineal-gland/*.

Lucas, R. J., G. S. Lall, and A. E. Allen. 2012. "How Rod, Cone, and Melanopsin Photoreceptors Come Together to Enlighten the Mammalian Circadian Clock." *Progress in Brain Research* 199: 1–18.

Luppi, P., O. Clement, and P. Fort. 2013. "Paradoxical (REM) Sleep Genesis by the Brainstem Is under Hypothalamic Control." *Current Opinion in Neurobiology* 23: 1–7.

Luthe, Wolfgang, ed. 1969. *Autogenic Therapy,* vol. 1. New York: Grune & Stratton.

Macey, P. M., R. Kumar, M. A. Woo, E. M. Valladares, F. L. Yan-Go, and R. M. Harper. 2008. "Brain Structural Changes in Obstructive Sleep Apnea." *Sleep* 31: 967–77.

Macnaughton, Ian, ed. 2004. *Body, Breath and Consciousness: A Somatics Anthology.* Berkeley, CA: North Atlantic Books.

Mander, B. A., S. M. Marks, J. W. Vogel, V. Rao, B. Lu, J. M. Saletin, S. Ancoli-Israel, W. J. Jagust, and M. P. Walker. 2015. "β-amyloid Disrupts Human NREM Slow Waves and Related Hippocampus-Dependent Memory Consolidation." *Nature Neuroscience* 18 (7): 1051–57.

Mander, B. A., S. Santhanam, and M. P. Walker. 2011. "Wake Deterioration and Sleep Restoration of Human Learning." *Current Biology* 21 (5): 183–84.

Mander, B. A., J. R. Winer, and M. P. Walker. 2017. "Sleep and Human Aging." *Neuron* 94 (1): 19–36.

McCall, Timothy. 2007. *Yoga as Medicine: The Yogic Prescription for Health and Healing*. New York: Bantam Dell.

McCarley, R. W. 2004. "Mechanisms and Models of REM Sleep Control." *Archives Italiennes de Biologie* 142: 429–67.

McCarley, R. W., J. W. Winkelman, and F. H. Duffy. 1983. "Human Cerebral Potentials Associated with REM Sleep Rapid Eye Movements: Links to PGO Waves and Waking Potentials." *Brain Research* 274: 359–64.

McKenna, B. S., D. L. Dickinson, H. J. Orff, and S. P. Drummond. 2007. "The Effects of One Night of Sleep Deprivation on Known-Risk and Ambiguous-Risk Decisions." *Journal of Sleep Research* 16: 245–52.

Mead, Alice. 2017. "The Legal Status of Cannabis (Marijuana) and Cannabidiol (CBD) under U.S. Law." *Epilepsy and Behavior* 70: 288–91.

Mechoulam, R., and L. Parker. 2013. "Towards a Better Cannabis Drug." *British Journal of Pharmacology* 170 (7): 1363–64.

Mechoulam, R., L. A. Parker, and R. Gallily. 2002. "Cannabidiol: An Overview of Some Pharmacological Aspects." *Journal of Clinical Pharmacology* 42 (Suppl. 11): 11S–19S.

Miller, Richard. 2005. *Yoga Nidra: A Meditative Practice for Deep Relaxation and Healing*. Boulder, CO: Sounds True.

Mindell, J. A., B. Kuhn, D. S. Lewin, L. J. Meltzer, and A. Sadeh. 2006. "Behavioral Treatment of Bedtime Problems and Night Wakings in Infants and Young Children." *Sleep* 29: 1263–76.

Monier-Williams, Monier. 1899. *A Sanskrit-English Dictionary: Etymologically and Philologically Arranged with Special Reference to Cognate Indo-European Languages*. Oxford: Clarendon Press.

Monk, T. H. 2005. "Aging Human Circadian Rhythms: Conventional Wisdom May Not Always Be Right." *Journal of Biological Rhythms* 20: 366–74.

Montgomery, I., J. Trinder, S. Paxton, G. Fraser, M. Meaney, and G. L. Koerbin. 1985. "Sleep Disruption Following a Marathon." *Journal of Sports Medicine and Physical Fitness* 25: 69–74.

Moore, R. Y. 1983. "Organization and Function of a Central Nervous System Circadian Oscillator: The Suprachiasmatic Nucleus." *Federation Proceedings* 42: 2783–89.

Morin, C. M., G. Belleville, L. Belanger, and H. Ivers. 2011. "The Insomnia Severity Index: Psychometric Indicators to Detect Insomnia Cases and Evaluate Treatment Response." *Sleep* 34: 601–8.

Morin, C. M., M. LeBlanc, M. Daley, J. P. Grégoire, and C. Mérette. 2006. "Epidemiology of Insomnia: Prevalence, Self-Help Treatments and Consultations Initiated, and Determinants of Help-Seeking Behaviors." *Sleep Medicine* 7: 123–30.

Mosqueda-Garcia, R., D. Robertson, and R. M. Robertson. 1993. "The Cardiovascular Effects of Caffeine." In *Caffeine, Coffee, and Health,* edited by S. Garattini, 157–76. New York: Raven.

Mustian, K. M. 2013. "Yoga as Treatment for Insomnia among Cancer Patients and Survivors: A Systematic Review." *European Medical Journal* 1: 106–15.

Muzet, A. 2007. "Environmental Noise, Sleep and Health." *Sleep Medicine Review* 11: 135–42.

Muzur, A., E. F. Pace-Schott, and J. A. Hobson. 2002. "The Prefrontal Cortex in Sleep." *Trends in Cognitive Science* 6: 475–81.

Myllymaki, T., H. Kyrolainen, K. Savolainen, L. Hokka, R. Jakonen, and T. Juuti. 2011. "Effects of Vigorous Late-Night Exercise on Sleep Quality and Cardiac Autonomic Activity." *Journal of Sleep Research* 20: 146–53.

Nakayama, M. 1991. "Histological Study on Aging Changes in the Human Tongue." *Nippon Jibiinkoka Gakkai Kaiho* 94: 541–55.

Nardi, A. E., F. L. Lopes, R. C. Freire, A. B. Veras, I. Nascimento, A. M. Valença, V. L. de-Melo-Neto, G. L. Soares-Filho, A. L. King, D. M. Araújo, M. A. Mezzasalma, A. Rassi, and W. A. Zin. 2009. "Panic Disorder and Social Anxiety Disorder Subtypes in a Caffeine Challenge Test." *Psychiatry Research* 169 (2): 149–53.

Neckelmann, D., A. Mykletun, and A. A. Dahl. 2007. "Chronic Insomnia as a Risk Factor for Developing Anxiety and Depression." *Sleep* 30: 873–80.

Nedergaard, M., and S. A. Goldman. 2016. "Brain Drain." *Scientific American* 314: 44–49.

Neikrug, A. B., and S. Ancoli-Israel. 2010. "Sleep Disorders in the Older Adult: A Mini-Review." *Gerontology* 56 (2): 181–89.

Odier, Daniel. 2005. *Yoga Spandakarika: The Sacred Texts at the Origins of Tantra.* Rochester, VT: Inner Traditions.

Ohayon, M. M., M. A. Carskadon, C. Guilleminault, and M. V. Vitiello. 2004. "Meta-analysis of Quantitative Sleep Parameters from Childhood to

Old Age in Healthy Individuals: Developing Normative Sleep Values across the Human Lifespan." *Sleep* 27 (7): 1255–73.

Ohayon, M. M., C. Guilleminault, and R. G. Priest. 1999. "Night Terrors, Sleepwalking, and Confusional Arousals in the General Population: Their Frequency and Relationship to Other Sleep and Mental Disorders." *Journal of Clinical Psychiatry* 60: 268–76.

Ohayon, M. M., and Charles F. Reynolds III. 2009. "Epidemiological and Clinical Relevance of Insomnia Diagnosis Algorithms according to the DSM-IV and the International Classification of Sleep Disorders (ICSD)." *Sleep Medicine* 10 (9): 952–60.

Ohayon, M. M., and T. Roth. 2002. "Prevalence of Restless Legs Syndrome and Periodic Limb Movement Disorder in the General Population." *Journal of Psychosomatic Research* 53: 547–54.

Okajima, I., Y. Komada, and Y. Inoue. 2011. "A Meta-analysis on the Treatment Effectiveness of Cognitive Behavioral Therapy for Primary Insomnia." *Sleep and Biological Rhythms* 9: 24–34.

Olff, M., J. L. Frijling, L. D. Kubzansky, B. Bradley, M. A. Ellenbogen, C. Cardoso, J. A. Bartz, J. R. Yee, and M. van Zuiden. 2013. "The Role of Oxytocin in Social Bonding, Stress Regulation and Mental Health: An Update on the Moderating Effects of Context and Interindividual Differences." *Psychoneuroendocrinology* 38 (9): 1883–94.

Ong, J. C., R. L. Shapiro, and R. Manber. 2008. "Combining Mindfulness Meditation with Cognitive-Behavior Therapy for Insomnia: A Treatment-Development Study." *Behavioral Therapy* 39: 171–82.

Papp, M. E. 2017. "Effects of Yogic Exercises on Functional Capacity, Lung Function and Quality of Life in Participants with Obstructive Pulmonary Disease: A Randomized Controlled Study." *European Journal of Physical and Rehabilitation Medicine* 53 (3): 447–61.

Payne, J. M. 2010. "Memory Consolidation, The Diurnal Rhythm of Cortisol, and the Nature of Dreams: A New Hypothesis." *International Review of Neurobiology* 92: 101–34.

Payne, P., and M. A. Crane-Godreau. 2015. "Meditative Movement for Depression and Anxiety." *Frontiers in Psychiatry* 4: 71.

Pearce, J. M. 1989. "Clinical Features of the Exploding Head Syndrome." *Journal of Neurological and Neurosurgical Psychiatry* 52: 907–10.

Peppard, P. E., and T. Young. 2004. "Exercise and Sleep-Disordered Breathing: An Association Independent of Body Habitus." *Sleep* 27 (3): 480–84.

Perlis, M. L., L. J. Smith, J. M. Lyness, S. R. Matteson, W. R. Pigeon, C. R. Jungquist, and X. Tu. 2006. "Insomnia as a Risk Factor for Onset of Depression in the Elderly." *Behavioral Sleep Medicine* 4 (2): 104–13.

Perls, Fritz. 1973. *The Gestalt Approach and Eye Witness to Therapy.* Mountain View, CA: Science Behavior Books.

Pilcher, J. J., and M. K. Coplen. 2000. "Work/Rest Cycles in Railroad Operations: Effects of Shorter Than 24-h Shift Work Schedules and On-call Schedules on Sleep." *Ergonomics* 43: 573–88.

Plante, D. T., and W. Winkelman. 2006. "Parasomnias." *Psychiatric Clinics of North America* 29: 969–87.

Plog, B., and M. Nedergaard. 2018. "The Glymphatic System in Central Nervous System Health and Disease: Past, Present, and Future." *Annual Review of Pathology* 13: 379–94.

Pressman, M. R. 2007. "Factors That Predispose, Prime and Precipitate NREM Parasomnias in Adults: Clinical and Forensic Implications." *Sleep Medicine Review* 11: 5–30.

Qualter, P., S. L. Brown, P. Munn, and K. J. Rotenberg. 2010. "Childhood Loneliness as a Predictor of Adolescent Depressive Symptoms: An 8-Year Longitudinal Study." *European Child and Adolescent Psychiatry* 19: 493–501.

Raichle, M. E., A. M. MacLeod, A. Z. Snyder, W. J. Powers, D. A. Gusnard, and G. L. Shulman. 2001. "A Default Mode of Brain Function." *Proceedings of the National Academy of Sciences of the United States of America* 98: 676–82.

Rama, Swami. 1976. *Yoga and Psychotherapy: The Evolution of Consciousness.* Honesdale, PA: Himalayan Institute.

Rechtschaffen, A., and A. Kales. 1968. *A Manual of Standardized Terminology, Techniques and Scoring System for Sleep Stages of Human Subjects.* Washington, DC: National Institutes of Health.

Rediehs, M. H., J. S. Reis, and N. S. Creason. 1990. "Sleep in Old Age: Focus on Gender Differences." *Sleep* 13 (5): 410–24.

Richardson, G. S., J. D. Miner, and C. A. Czeisler. 1989. "Impaired Driving Performance in Shiftworkers: The Role of the Circadian System in a Multifactorial Model." *Alcohol, Drugs and Driving* 5–6: 265–73.

Roebuck, Valerie, trans. and ed. 2003. *The Upanishads.* London: Penguin Books.

Roehrs, T., and T. Roth. 2001. "Sleep, Sleepiness, and Alcohol Use." *Alcohol Research & Health* 25: 101–9.

Roenneberg, T. 2007. "Epidemiology of the Human Circadian Clock." *Sleep Medicine Review* 11: 429–38.

Roenneberg, T., A. Wirz-Justice, and M. Merrow. 2003. "Life between Clocks: Daily Temporal Patterns of Human Chronotypes." *Journal of Biological Rhythms* 18: 80–90.

Rogers, G. S., R. L. Van de Castle, W. S. Evans, and J. W. Critelli. 1985. "Vaginal Pulse Amplitude Response Patterns during Erotic Conditions and Sleep." *Archives of Sexual Behavior* 14: 327–42.

Saper, C. B., G. Cano, and T. E. Scammell. 2005. "Homeostatic, Circadian, and Emotional Regulation of Sleep." *Journal of Comparative Neurology* 493: 92–98.

Saper, C. B., T. E. Scammell, and J. Lu. 2005. "Hypothalamic Regulation of Sleep and Circadian Rhythms." *Nature* 437: 1257–63.

Sapienza, C., M. Troche, T. Pitts, and P. Davenport. 2011. "Respiratory Strength Training: Concept and Intervention Outcomes." *Seminars in Speech and Language* 32: 21–30.

Satyananda Saraswati, Swami. 1976. *Yoga Nidra.* Munger, Bihar, India: Yoga Publications Trust.

Scammell, T. E. 2003. "The Neurobiology, Diagnosis, and Treatment of Narcolepsy." *Annals of Neurology* 53: 154–66.

Schenck, C. H., S. R. Bundlie, M. G. Ettinger, and M. W. Mahowald. 1986. "Chronic Behavioral Disorders of Human REM Sleep: A New Category of Parasomnia." *Sleep* 9: 293–308.

Schwartz, M. D., and T. D. Kilduff. 2015. "The Neurobiology of Sleep and Wakefulness." *Psychiatric Clinics of North America* 38 (4): 615–44.

Seeman, M. V. 2011. "Sleepwalking: A Possible Side Effect of Antipsychotic Medication." *Psychiatry Quarterly* 82: 59–67.

Shamsuzzaman, A. S., B. J. Gersh, and V. K. Somers. 2003. "Obstructive Sleep Apnea: Implications for Cardiac and Vascular Disease." *Journal of the American Medical Association* 290: 1906–14.

Shapiro, C. M., R. Bortz, D. Mitchell, R. A. Clarke, and P. L. Jooste. 1985. "Effect of Exercise in a Hot Environment on Human Sleep Patterns." *South African Journal of Science* 81: 624–27.

Sharma, Arvind. 2004. *Sleep as a State of Consciousness in Advaita Vedānta.* Albany: State University of New York Press.

Sharpless, B. A., and J. P. Barber. 2011. "Lifetime Prevalence Rates of Sleep Paralysis: A Systematic Review." *Sleep Medicine Reviews* 15 (5): 311–15.

Shochat, T., J. Martin, M. Marler, and S. Ancoli-Israel. 2000. "Illumination Levels in Nursing Home Patients: Effects on Sleep and Activity Rhythms." *Journal of Sleep Research* 9 (4): 373–80.

Shusterman, Richard. 2008. *Body Consciousness: A Philosophy of Mindfulness and Somaesthetics*. New York: Cambridge University Press.

Shusterman, Richard. 2012. *Thinking through the Body: Essays in Somaesthetics*. New York: Cambridge University Press.

Siclari, F., R. Khatami, and F. Urbaniok. 2010. "Violence in Sleep." *Brain* 133: 3494–95.

Singareddy, R. K., and R. Balon. 2002. "Sleep in Posttraumatic Stress Disorder." *Annals of Clinical Psychiatry* 14: 183–90.

Singh, S., K. Singh, S. P. Gupta, D. K. Patel, V. K. Singh, R. K. Singh, and M. P. Singh. 2009. "Effect of Caffeine on the Expression of Cytochrome P450 1A2, Adenosine A2A Receptor and Dopamine Transporter in Control and 1-methyl 4-phenyl 1, 2, 3, 6-tetrahydropyridine Treated Mouse Striatum." *Brain Research* 1283: 115–26.

Slavich, G. M., and M. R. Irwin. 2014. "From Stress to Inflammation and Major Depressive Disorder: A Social Signal Transduction Theory of Depression." *Psychological Bulletin* 140 (3): 774–815.

Smets, E. M. 1995. "Multidimensional Fatigue Inventory (MFI): Psychometric Qualities of an Instrument to Assess Fatigue." *Journal of Psychosomatic Research* 39 (3): 315–25.

Smith, M. T., and J. A. Haythornthwaite. 2004. "How Do Sleep Disturbance and Chronic Pain Inter-relate? Insights from the Longitudinal and Cognitive Behavioral Clinical Trials Literature." *Sleep Medicine Review* 8: 119–32.

Sobrinho, L. G. 2003. "Prolactin, Psychological Stress and Environment in Humans: Adaptation and Maladaptation." *Pituitary* 6 (1): 35–39.

Spiegel, K., E. Tasali, R. Leproult, and E. Van Cauter. 2009. "Effects of Poor and Short Sleep on Glucose Metabolism and Obesity Risk." *National Review of Endocrinology* 5: 253–61.

Spielberger, C. D. 1983. *Manual for the State-Trait Anxiety Inventory (STAI)*. Palo Alto, CA: Consulting Psychologists Press.

Spielberger, C. D., R. L. Gorsuch, and R. E. Lushene. 1970. *Manual for the State-Trait Anxiety Inventory*. Palo Alto, CA: California Consulting Psychologists Press.

St.-Onge, M. P., A. Roberts, A. Shechter, and A. R. Choudhury. 2016. "Fiber and Saturated Fat Are Associated with Sleep Arousals and Slow Wave Sleep." *Journal of Clinical Sleep Medicine* 12: 19–24.

Stein, M. D., and P. D. Friedmann. 2005. "Disturbed Sleep and Its Relationship to Alcohol Use." *Substance Abuse* 26: 1–13.

Stephens, Mark. 2010. *Teaching Yoga: Essential Foundations, Principles, and Techniques.* Berkeley, CA: North Atlantic Books.

Stephens, Mark. 2012. *Yoga Sequencing: Designing Transformative Yoga Classes.* Berkeley, CA: North Atlantic Books.

Stephens, Mark. 2014. *Yoga Adjustments: Philosophy, Principles, and Techniques.* Berkeley, CA: North Atlantic Books.

Stephens, Mark. 2017. *Yoga Therapy: Foundations, Methods, and Practices for Common Ailments.* Berkeley, CA: North Atlantic Books.

Steriade, M. M., and R. W. McCarley. 2005. *Brain Control of Wakefulness and Sleep.* New York: Kluwer Academic/Plenum.

Storandt, M., E. A. Grant, J. P. Miller, and J. C. Morris. 2006. "Longitudinal Course and Neuropathologic Outcomes in Original vs. Revised MCI and in Pre-MCI." *Neurology* 67 (3): 467–73.

Stores, G. 2003. "Medication for Sleep-Wake Disorders." *Archives of Disease in Childhood* 88: 899–903.

Stores, G. 2006. "Sleep Disorders." In *A Clinician's Handbook of Childhood and Adolescent Psychiatry,* edited by C. Gillberg, R. Harrington, and H. C. Steinhausen, 304–38. Cambridge: Cambridge University Press.

Stores, G. 2007. "Parasomnias of Childhood and Adolescence." *Sleep Medicine Clinics* 2: 405–17.

Stores, G. 2008. *Sleep Problems in Children and Adolescents: The Facts.* Oxford: Oxford University Press.

Stores, G. 2009. "Aspects of Sleep Disorders in Children and Adolescents." *Dialogues in Clinical Neuroscience* 11 (1): 87.

Stranges, S., J. M. Dorn, and F. P. Cappuccio. 2010. "A Population-Based Study of Reduced Sleep Duration and Hypertension: The Strongest Association May Be in Premenopausal Women." *Journal of Hypertension* 28: 896–902.

Stranges, S., W. Tigbe, F. X. Gómez-Olivé, M. Thorogood, and N. B. Kandala. 2012. "Sleep Problems: An Emerging Global Epidemic?" *Sleep* 35 (8): 1173–81.

Swaab, D. F., E. Fliers, and T. S. Partiman. 1985. "The Suprachiasmatic Nucleus of the Human Brain in Relation to Sex, Age and Senile Dementia." *Brain Research* 342: 37–44.

Swatmarama, Swami. 1985. *Hatha Yoga Pradipika.* Edited by Swami Muktibodhananda. Munger, Bihar, India: Yoga Publications Trust.

Takahashi, S., T. Ono, Y. Ishiwata, and T. Kuroda. 2002. "Breathing Modes, Body Positions, and Suprahyoid Muscle Activity." *Journal of Orthodontics* 29: 307–13.

Tang, N. K. Y. 2008. "Insomnia Co-occurring with Chronic Pain: Clinical Features, Interaction, Assessments and Possible Interventions." *Review of Pain* 2: 2–7.

Taylor, D. J., O. G. Jenni, C. Acebo, and M. A. Carskadon. 2005. "Sleep Tendency during Extended Wakefulness: Insights into Adolescent Sleep Regulation and Behavior." *Journal of Sleep Research* 14: 239–44.

Thase, M. E., J. B. Greenhouse, and E. Frank. 1997. "Treatment of Major Depression with Psychotherapy or Psychotherapy-Pharmacotherapy Combinations." *Archives of General Psychiatry* 54 (11): 1009–15.

Thornton, H. R., J. Miller, L. Taylor, C. Sargent, M. Lastella, and P. M. Fowler. 2017. "Impact of Short- Compared to Long-Haul International Travel on the Sleep and Wellbeing of National Wheelchair Basketball Athletes." *Journal of Sports Science* 3: 1–9.

Todd, Mabel. 1937. *The Thinking Body: A Study of the Balancing Forces of Dynamic Man.* Gouldsboro, ME: Gestalt Journal Press.

Touitou, Y. 2001. "Human Aging and Melatonin: Clinical Relevance." *Experimental Gerontology* 36 (7): 1083–1100.

U.S. Centers for Disease Control and Prevention. 2014. "Short Sleep Duration among U.S. Adults." Table 1. *www.cdc.gov/sleep/data_statistics.html.*

U.S. Centers for Disease Control and Prevention. 2018. "Suicide Rising across the U.S." *www.cdc.gov/vitalsigns/suicide/index.html.*

U.S. Centers for Disease Control and Prevention. 2019. "U.S. Opioid Prescribing Rate Maps." *www.cdc.gov/drugoverdose/maps/rxrate-maps.html.*

U.S. Congress. 2019. "H. R. 2—Agriculture Improvement Act of 2018." 115th Congress (2017–18). *www.congress.gov/bill/115th-congress/house-bill/2/text.*

U.S. National Institutes of Health. 2015. "Tips for Getting a Good Night's Sleep." *NIH MedlinePlus* 10 (2): 22. *https://medlineplus.gov/magazine/issues/summer15/articles/summer15pg22.html.*

van der Helm, E., N. Gujar, C. Watts, and M. P. Walker. 2010. "Sleep Deprivation Impairs the Ability to Recognize Human Emotions." *Sleep* 33: 335–42.

Van der Kolk, K. B. 1984. "Nightmares and Trauma: A Comparison of Nightmares after Combat with Lifelong Nightmares in Veterans." *American Journal of Psychiatry* 141: 187–90.

Van der Kolk, K. B. 2014. *The Body Keeps Score: Brain, Mind, and Body in the Healing of Trauma.* New York: Penguin Books.

van Lutterveld, R., E. van Dellen, P. Pal, H. Yang, C. J. Stam, and J. Brewer. 2017. "Meditation Is Associated with Increased Brain Network Integration." *NeuroImage* 158: 18–25.

Varela, F., E. Rosch, and E. Thompson. 2016. *The Embodied Mind: Cognitive Science and Human Experience.* Cambridge, MA: MIT Press.

Venkatraman, V., Y. M. Chuah, S. A. Huettel, and M. W. Chee. 2007. "Sleep Deprivation Elevates Expectation of Gains and Attenuates Response to Losses Following Risky Decisions." *Sleep* 30: 603–9.

Vinters, H. V. 2015. "Emerging Concepts in Alzheimer's Disease." *Annual Review of Pathology* 10: 291–319.

Vitiello, M. V. 1996. "Sleep Disorders and Aging." *Current Opinion in Psychiatry* 9 (4): 284–89.

Wahlstrom, K. L., and J. A. Owens. 2017. "School Start Time Effects on Adolescent Learning and Academic Performance, Emotional Health and Behaviour." *Current Opinion in Psychiatry* 30 (6): 485–90.

Walker, M. P. 2008. "Cognitive Consequences of Sleep and Sleep Loss." *Sleep Medicine* 9: S29–S34.

Walker, M. P. 2009. "The Role of Sleep in Cognition and Emotion." *Annals of the New York Academy of Sciences* 1156: 168–97.

Walker, Matthew. 2017. *Why We Sleep: Unlocking the Power of Sleep and Dreams.* New York: Scribner.

Walker, M. P., T. Brakefield, A. Morgan, J. A. Hobson, and R. Stickgold. 2002. "Practice Then Sleep Makes Perfect: Sleep Dependent Motor Skill Learning." *Neuron* 35 (1): 205–11.

Walker, M. P., and R. Stickgold. 2006. "Sleep, Memory, and Plasticity." *Annual Review of Psychology* 57: 139–66.

Walsh, R., and S. L. Shapiro. 2006. "The Meeting of Meditative Disciplines and Western Psychology: A Mutually Enriching Dialogue." *American Psychologist* 61 (3): 227–39.

Ware, J., Jr., M. Kosinski, and S. D. Keller. 1996. "A 12-Item Short-Form Health Survey: Construction of Scales and Preliminary Tests of Reliability and Validity." *Medical Care* 34 (3): 220–33.

Wehrle, R., C. Kaufmann, T. C. Wetter, F. Holsboer, D. P. Auer, T. Poll-mächer, and M. Czisch. 2007. "Functional Microstates within Human REM Sleep: First Evidence from fMRI of a Thalamocortical Network Specific for Phasic REM Periods." *European Journal of Neuroscience* 25: 863–71.

Weintraub, Amy. 2004. *Yoga for Depression: A Compassionate Guide to Relieve Suffering through Yoga.* New York: Broadway.

Weissman, S., and R. Weissman. 1996. *Meditation, Compassion and Loving Kindness: An Approach to Vipassana Practice.* York Beach, ME: Weiser.

White, D. P. 2005. "Pathogenesis of Obstructive and Central Sleep Apnea." *American Journal of Respiratory Critical Care Medicine* 172: 1363–70.

White, David G., ed. 2012a. *Yoga in Practice.* Oxford: Oxford University Press.

White, David G. 2012b. *The Yoga Sutra of Patanjali: A Biography.* Oxford: Oxford University Press.

Wiegand, M. H., Z. Veselý, V. Krumbholz, J. Kronseder, and S. Diplich. 2002. "Antidepressant Effect of Sleep Deprivation: Relationship with Spontaneous Sleep Episodes." *Journal of Sleep Research* 11 (Suppl. 1): 251.

Wiggs, L. 2009. "Behavioural Aspects of Children's Sleep." *Archives of Disease in Childhood* 94: 59–62.

Wilcox, S., G. A. Brenes, D. Levine, M. A. Sevick, S. A. Shumaker, and T. Craven. 2000. "Factors related to Sleep Disturbance in Older Adults Experiencing Knee Pain or Knee Pain with Radiographic Evidence of Knee Osteoarthritis." *Journal of the American Geriatrics Society* 48 (10): 1241–51.

Wilkins, W. J. 2003. *Hindu Gods and Goddesses.* Mineola, NY: Dover.

Wilson, A. G. 2017. "Why Sex Is Good for Sleep: Adelaide Sleep Researcher Dr. Michele Lastella Explains." *The Advertiser,* December 3. *www .adelaidenow.com.au/lifestyle/relationships/why-sex-is-good-for-sleep -adelaide-sleep-researcher-dr-michele-lastella-explains/news-story/.*

Wilson, S. J. 2010. "British Association for Psychopharmacology Consensus Statement on Evidence-Based Treatment of Insomnia, Parasomnias and Circadian Rhythm Disorders." *Journal of Psychopharmacology* 24 (11): 1577–1601.

Winter, W. Chris. 2017. *The Sleep Solution: Why Your Sleep Is Broken and How to Fix It.* New York: Berkley.

Wolfson, A. R., and M. A. Carskadon. 2003. "Understanding Adolescents' Sleep Patterns and School Performance: A Critical Appraisal." *Sleep Medicine Review* 7: 491–506.

Woods, James Haughton, trans. 2003. *The Yoga Sutras of Patañjali.* Mineola, NY: Courier Dover Publications.

Young, T., M. Palta, J. Dempsey, J. Skatrud, S. Weber, and S. Badr. 1993. "The Occurrence of Sleep-Disordered Breathing among Middle-Aged Adults." *New England Journal of Medicine* 328: 1230–35.

Young, T., D. Rabago, A. Zgierska, D. Austin, and L. Finn. 2003. "Objective and Subjective Sleep Quality in Premenopausal, Perimenopausal, and Postmenopausal Women in the Wisconsin Sleep Study." *Sleep* 26: 667–72.

Youngstedt, S. D. 2005. "Effects of Exercise on Sleep." *Clinical Sports Medicine* 24: 355–65.

Yumino, D., H. Wang, J. S. Floras, G. E. Newton, S. Mak, P. Ruttanaumpawan, J. D. Parker, and T. D. Bradley. 2009. "Prevalence and Physiological Predictors of Sleep Apnea in Patients with Heart Failure and Systolic Dysfunction." *Journal of Cardiac Failure* 15: 279–85.

Yurtkuran, M., A. Alp, and K. Dilek. 2007. "A Modified Yoga-Based Exercise Program in Hemodialysis Patients: A Randomized Controlled Study." *Complementary and Therapeutic Medicine* 15: 164–71.

Zeitzer, J. M., D. J. Dijk, R. Kronauer, E. Brown, and C. Czeisler. 2000. "Sensitivity of the Human Circadian Pacemaker to Nocturnal Light: Melatonin Phase Resetting and Suppression." *Journal of Physiology* 526 (Part 3): 695–702.

INDEX

N

ABOUT THE AUTHOR

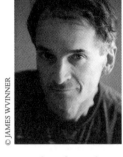

MARK STEPHENS is the author of four best-selling books for yoga teachers and therapists: *Teaching Yoga* (2010), *Yoga Sequencing* (2012), *Yoga Adjustments* (2014), and *Yoga Therapy* (2017), as well as The Mark Stephens Yoga Sequencing Deck (2016). Practicing yoga daily since 1991 and teaching since 1996, Stephens is a yoga innovator who blends insights from human physiology, kinesiology, neuroscience, and psychosomatics with ancient to modern yoga and contemporary philosophies of consciousness and being. He lives in the Santa Cruz Mountains along the central coast of California and teaches yoga locally and globally. Learn more at *www.markstephensyoga.com*.

ALSO BY MARK STEPHENS

available from North Atlantic Books

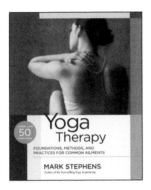

Yoga Therapy
978-1-62317-106-3

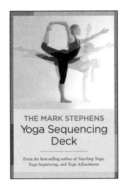

*The Mark Stephens
Yoga Sequencing Deck*
978-1-62317-061-5

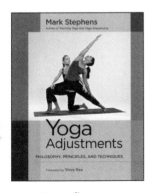

Yoga Adjustments
978-1-58394-770-8

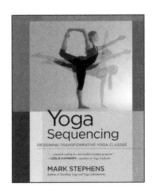

Yoga Sequencing
978-1-58394-497-4

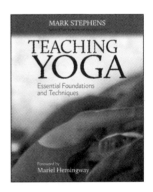

Teaching Yoga
978-1-55643-885-1

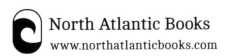 North Atlantic Books
www.northatlanticbooks.com

North Atlantic Books is an independent, nonprofit publisher committed to a bold exploration of the relationships between mind, body, spirit, and nature.

About North Atlantic Books

North Atlantic Books (NAB) is an independent, nonprofit publisher committed to a bold exploration of the relationships between mind, body, spirit, and nature. Founded in 1974, NAB aims to nurture a holistic view of the arts, sciences, humanities, and healing. To make a donation or to learn more about our books, authors, events, and newsletter, please visit www.northatlanticbooks.com.

North Atlantic Books is the publishing arm of the Society for the Study of Native Arts and Sciences, a 501(c)(3) nonprofit educational organization that promotes cross-cultural perspectives linking scientific, social, and artistic fields. To learn how you can support us, please visit our website.